HASHIMOTO'S HEALING WORKBOOK

A 12-Week Plan to Heal Your Thyroiditis: Lose Weight, Balance Hormones, Restore Energy, and Eliminate Chronic Fatigue

Emma Jane Harper

© 2024 Hashimoto's Healing Workbook. Emma Jane Harper. All rights reserved. This book is for informational use only. It is provided "as is" without any warranties, either express or implied. The publisher assumes no responsibility for any damages arising from the use or misuse of the information contained herein. Unauthorized reproduction, distribution, or transmission of this book, in whole or in part, is strictly prohibited. All trademarks and brand names mentioned are the property of their respective owners.

Table of Contents

CHAPTER 1: WELCOME TO YOUR HEALING JOURNEY 7
    1.1: What Is Hashimoto's? Understanding the Condition 7
    1.2: Why This Workbook Was Created 9
    1.3: My Personal Experience with Hashimoto's 10

PART 1: UNDERSTANDING HASHIMOTO'S AND THYROIDITIS 13

CHAPTER 2: THYROID HEALTH 101 14
    2.1: The Role of the Thyroid 14
    2.2: Autoimmunity in Hashimoto's Explained 16
    2.3: Common Symptoms and Misdiagnoses 18
    2.4: Root Causes of Thyroiditis: Gut, Inflammation, Stress 20

CHAPTER 3: THE HASHIMOTO'S VICIOUS CYCLE 22
    3.1: Inflammation, Hormones, and Lifestyle Factors 22
    3.2: Breaking the Cycle: A New Approach to Healing 24

CHAPTER 4: MYTHS AND MISCONCEPTIONS ABOUT HASHIMOTO'S 26
    4.1: Debunking Myths About Diet, Medication, and Healing 26
    4.2: The Truth About Levothyroxine and Medications 28
    4.3: Symptom Management vs. Root Cause Healing 30

PART 2: PREPARING FOR SUCCESS 32

CHAPTER 5: PREPARING FOR YOUR 12-WEEK PLAN 33
    5.1: Setting Realistic Expectations 33
    5.2 Workbook Exercise: Writing Your Health Vision Statement 35

CHAPTER 6: ESSENTIAL TOOLS FOR HEALING 37
    6.1: Supplements, Lab Tests, and Resources 37
    6.2: Using Symptom Trackers and Food Journals 40
    6.3 Workbook Exercise: Tracking Your Current Baseline (Energy, Mood, Symptoms) 42

PART 3: THE 12-WEEK HEALING PLAN 44

CHAPTER 7: RESET AND DETOX 45

  7.1: Eliminating Gluten, Dairy, Sugar, and Processed Foods 45
   Detox Recipe 1: Green Smoothie 46
   Detox Recipe 2: Turmeric Ginger Tea 47
   Detox Recipe 3: Quinoa Salad 47
  7.2: Supporting Liver Health for Detoxification 48
   Detox Beverage Recipes: 49
  7.3 Workbook Exercise: Daily Food Tracker and Detox Checklist 51

CHAPTER 8: REBUILD AND NOURISH 53
  8.1: Incorporating Anti-Inflammatory Foods 53
   Turmeric Chicken & Vegetables 54
   Salmon with Avocado Salsa 55
   Spinach and Berry Smoothie 56
  8.2: Key Nutrients for Thyroid Function 57
   Recipe 1: Brazil Nut Smoothie 57
   Recipe 2: Seared Scallops with Mushroom Sauce 57
   Recipe 1: Pumpkin Seed Pesto 58
   Recipe 2: Beef and Lentil Stew 58
   Recipe 1: Salmon with Lemon and Dill 59
   Recipe 2: Spinach and Mushroom Omelet 59
  8.3 Workbook Exercise: Weekly Meal Planning 60

CHAPTER 9: GUT HEALTH AND HORMONAL BALANCE 62
  9.1: Healing the Gut with Probiotics and Enzymes 62
   Fermented Carrot and Ginger Salad 63
   Pineapple Papaya Smoothie 64
   Kefir Overnight Oats 65
  9.2: Reducing Cortisol and Supporting Adrenal Health 66
   Ashwagandha Moon Milk 66
   Salmon Avocado Salad 67
  9.3 Workbook Exercise: Tracking Digestive Changes 68

CHAPTER 10: ENERGY RESTORATION IN WEEKS 7-8 70
  10.1: Combating Fatigue with Sleep, Movement, and Hydration 70
   1. Berry Chia Seed Pudding 71

    2. Spinach and Mushroom Omelette 72

    3. Quinoa Breakfast Bowl 72

    10.2 Workbook Exercise: Energy Tracker and Self-Care Planner 73

CHAPTER 11: LONG-TERM MAINTENANCE 75

    11.1: Reintroducing Foods and Monitoring Reactions 75

    11.2: Building Resilience Against Relapses 77

        Sustainable Salmon Quinoa Salad 78

        Anti-Inflammatory Turmeric Chicken and Vegetables 79

    11.3 Workbook Exercise: Reflection and Setting Goals 80

PART 4: ADVANCED TOOLS AND RESOURCES 82

CHAPTER 12: NUTRITION AND DIETARY GUIDANCE 83

    12.1: Introducing Anti-Inflammatory Foods 83

        Recipe 1: Omega-3 Rich Salmon with Garlic Spinach 85

        Recipe 2: Anti-Inflammatory Berry Smoothie 85

        Recipe 3: Turmeric Ginger Tea 86

    12.2: Cooking Without Inflammatory Oils 87

        Recipe 1: Avocado Oil Roasted Brussels Sprouts 88

        Recipe 2: Coconut Oil Stir-Fry with Vegetables and Chicken 89

    12.3: Anti-Inflammatory Spices 90

        Golden Turmeric Latte 91

        Anti-Inflammatory Smoothie Bowl 91

CHAPTER 13: NUTRITIONAL BUILDING BLOCKS FOR THYROID HEALTH 93

    13.1: Selenium-Rich Foods 93

        Recipe 1: Selenium-Boosting Snack Mix 95

        Recipe 2: Simple Tuna and Avocado Salad 95

    13.2: Zinc-Rich Foods and Recipes 96

        Recipe 1: Zinc-Boosting Beef Stir-Fry 97

        Recipe 2: Lentil and Spinach Salad 98

    13.3: Vitamin D and Iodine Sources 99

        Recipe 1: Salmon with Roasted Vegetables 99

        Recipe 2: Seaweed Salad with Sesame Dressing 100

CHAPTER 14: GUT HEALTH AND HORMONAL BALANCE 101

14.1: Probiotic Foods and Digestive Enzymes 101
- Recipe 1: Probiotic-Rich Yogurt Bowl 102
- Recipe 2: Homemade Sauerkraut 103
- Recipe 3: Kefir Smoothie 103

14.2: Foods for Cortisol Management and Balanced Meals 104
- Recipe 1: Omega-3 Rich Salmon Salad 105
- Recipe 2: Stress-Reducing Berry Smoothie 105

CHAPTER 15: RECIPES AND MEAL PLANNING TOOLS 107

15.1: Easy Breakfast Recipes 107
- Recipe 1: Simple Avocado Toast 107
- Recipe 2: Quick Oatmeal with Berries 108
- Recipe 3: Easy Greek Yogurt Parfait 110
- Recipe 4: Basic Smoothie Bowl 111
- Recipe 5: Classic Scrambled Eggs 113

15.2: Easy Lunch Recipes 114
- Recipe 6: Grilled Chicken Salad 114
- Recipe 7: Veggie Wrap with Hummus 116
- Recipe 8: Quinoa and Black Bean Bowl 117
- Recipe 9: Turkey and Avocado Sandwich 119
- Recipe 10: Lentil Soup 120

15.2 Easy Recipes for Dinner 122
- Recipe 11: Baked Salmon with Asparagus 122
- Recipe 12: Chicken Stir Fry with Vegetables 124
- Recipe 13: Spaghetti Squash with Marinara Sauce 125
- Recipe 14: Stuffed Bell Peppers 127
- Recipe 15: Zucchini Noodles with Pesto 129

15.3: 7-Day Meal Plan Examples 130

Chapter 1: Welcome to Your Healing Journey

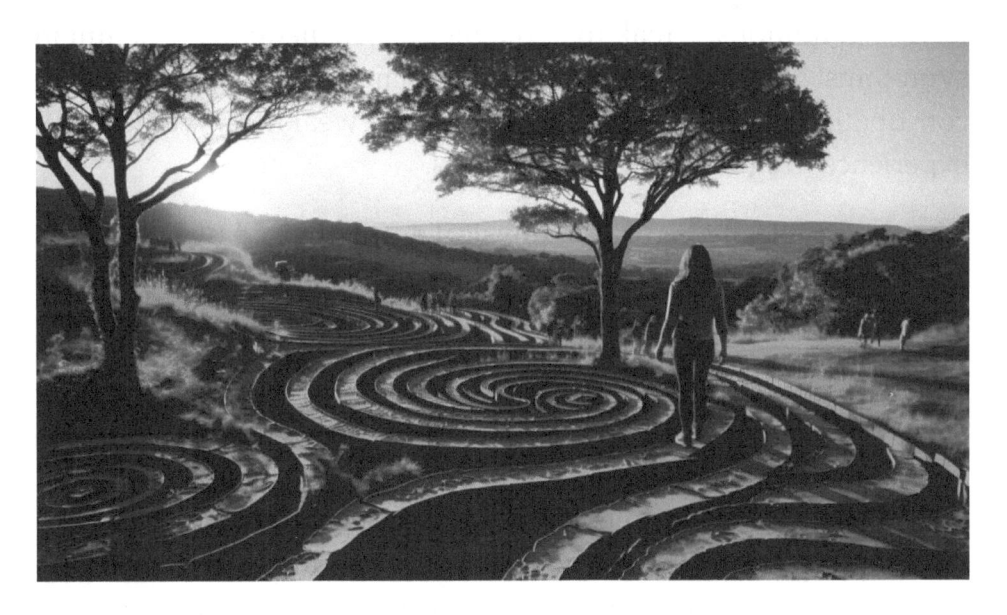

1.1: WHAT IS HASHIMOTO'S? UNDERSTANDING THE CONDITION

Hashimoto's, also known as Hashimoto's thyroiditis, is an autoimmune disorder where the immune system turns against the body's own tissues. In this case, it attacks the thyroid gland, a small butterfly-shaped gland located at the base of your neck. This gland plays a crucial role in regulating your metabolism through the release of hormones. When Hashimoto's disease affects the thyroid, it can lead to a reduction in hormone production, a condition known as hypothyroidism.

The exact cause of Hashimoto's is not fully understood, but it is believed to involve a combination of genetic and environmental factors. For instance, individuals with a family history of thyroid disorders are at higher risk. Environmental triggers may include excessive iodine intake, radiation exposure, and certain medications.

Symptoms of Hashimoto's can vary widely from person to person and may develop slowly over years. They often resemble those of other conditions, making diagnosis challenging. Common symptoms include fatigue, weight gain, sensitivity to cold, constipation, dry skin, hair loss, and muscle weakness. Women may experience irregular menstrual periods.

Diagnosis typically involves a physical exam, thyroid function tests, and antibody tests to detect the presence of thyroid peroxidase antibodies (TPOAb), which are found in the majority of Hashimoto's cases. These antibodies indicate an autoimmune attack on the thyroid.

Managing Hashimoto's focuses on restoring normal thyroid hormone levels. Treatment usually involves synthetic thyroid hormone replacement therapy, which requires careful monitoring by a healthcare provider to ensure correct dosage. Additionally, addressing lifestyle factors such as diet, stress, and exercise can help manage symptoms and improve overall well-being.

It's also important to be aware of the potential complications associated with untreated Hashimoto's, including heart problems, mental health issues, and complications during pregnancy. Therefore, early detection and treatment are crucial for preventing these outcomes and maintaining a high quality of life.

For those living with Hashimoto's, understanding the condition is the first step toward healing. Recognizing the symptoms, knowing the diagnostic process, and being informed about treatment options empowers individuals to take an active role in their health care journey. With the right approach, it is possible to manage Hashimoto's effectively and lead a healthy, fulfilling life.

1.2: WHY THIS WORKBOOK WAS CREATED

This workbook emerges from a deep understanding that individuals grappling with Hashimoto's thyroiditis face a unique set of challenges. The condition, characterized by an autoimmune attack on the thyroid gland, can lead to a bewildering array of symptoms, from weight fluctuations and fatigue to hormonal imbalances and chronic pain. Despite these obstacles, the path to improved health and well-being is not only possible but achievable with the right guidance and resources. That is the foundational belief that has led to the creation of this comprehensive 12-week plan. It is designed to serve as a beacon of hope and a practical tool for those who have been navigating the often turbulent waters of thyroid health issues.

The primary goal of this workbook is to offer a structured, step-by-step approach to healing. Recognizing the complexity of Hashimoto's, it seeks to demystify the condition by providing clear, actionable strategies that address both the symptoms and the root causes. By focusing on dietary changes, lifestyle adjustments, and stress management techniques, this plan aims to rebalance hormones, reduce inflammation, and restore energy levels. It acknowledges the interconnectedness of the body's systems and emphasizes the importance of holistic healing practices.

Moreover, this workbook is rooted in the principle that knowledge is power. It endeavors to educate readers about the intricacies of their condition, empowering them with the information they need to make informed decisions about their health. Through a combination of scientific research, expert insights, and personal anecdotes, it offers a comprehensive overview of Hashimoto's thyroiditis, including its potential triggers, common misconceptions, and the latest treatment options.

Another key aspect of this workbook is its emphasis on personalization. Recognizing that Hashimoto's affects each individual differently, it encourages readers to become active participants in their healing journey. Through a series of workbook exercises, readers are invited to track their symptoms, identify their triggers, and reflect on their progress. These activities are designed to foster a deeper connection with one's body, enabling readers to tailor the healing plan to their unique needs and preferences.

In essence, this workbook was created as a response to the need for a more compassionate, comprehensive, and accessible resource for individuals living with Hashimoto's. It is a testament to the belief that, with the right support and guidance, healing is within reach. Whether you are newly diagnosed or have been managing your condition for years, this workbook offers a fresh perspective on Hashimoto's and equips you with the tools you need to reclaim your health and vitality.

1.3: My Personal Experience with Hashimoto's

Discovering that I had Hashimoto's was a pivotal moment in my life, one that brought both challenges and profound insights. My journey began with a series of symptoms that, for years, seemed unrelated and inexplicable. I was constantly fatigued, no matter how much I slept, and my weight fluctuated wildly without any clear reason. My hair thinned, and my skin became dry and lackluster. These physical changes were accompanied by mood swings and a pervasive sense of malaise that I couldn't shake off. Like many of you, I visited numerous doctors, each offering a different perspective, but none could pinpoint exactly what was wrong.

The diagnosis of Hashimoto's came as both a shock and a relief. Finally, there was a name for what I was experiencing, a validation of my symptoms that I wasn't imagining them. However, the diagnosis was just the beginning of a long road toward healing. I delved into research, seeking to understand this condition that had taken over my life. I learned that Hashimoto's is an autoimmune disorder where the immune system mistakenly attacks the thyroid, impairing its ability to produce hormones essential for metabolism and energy.

Armed with this knowledge, I embarked on a journey to reclaim my health. It became clear that conventional medicine, while necessary, was not sufficient on its own. I needed to make significant lifestyle changes. This meant revamping my diet to eliminate gluten, dairy, and processed foods, which are known to contribute to inflammation and autoimmunity. I incorporated foods rich in selenium, zinc, and vitamin D, nutrients vital for thyroid function and immune support.

Stress management became a non-negotiable part of my daily routine. I explored various techniques, from yoga and meditation to deep-breathing exercises and spending time in nature, to find what worked best for me. I also learned the importance of quality sleep and made it a priority to get at least eight hours of restful sleep each night.

Perhaps one of the most challenging aspects of this journey was learning to listen to my body and recognize the signs it was giving me. This meant slowing down and making self-care a priority, something that was foreign to me in my previously fast-paced life. It was a process of trial and error, learning what alleviated my symptoms and what made them worse. Through this process, I became attuned to my body's needs, learning to give it the nourishment, rest, and care it required.

My journey with Hashimoto's has taught me the power of resilience and the importance of advocating for one's health. It has shown me that healing is not linear, but a series of steps forward, sometimes

Chapter 1:
Welcome to Your Healing Journey

with steps back, and that's okay. Each step has been a learning opportunity, a chance to grow and understand my body better. While I still have days that are more challenging than others, I now have the tools and knowledge to navigate these moments.

To those of you embarking on this journey, know that you are not alone. Healing from Hashimoto's is possible with patience, perseverance, and a willingness to make changes. It requires a holistic approach, addressing not just the physical symptoms but the emotional and spiritual aspects of your well-being. This workbook is designed to guide you through this process, offering practical advice and strategies based on both scientific research and personal experience. Together, we can take steps toward healing and reclaim the vibrant health we deserve.

Part 1:
Understanding Hashimoto's and Thyroiditis

Chapter 2:
Thyroid Health 101

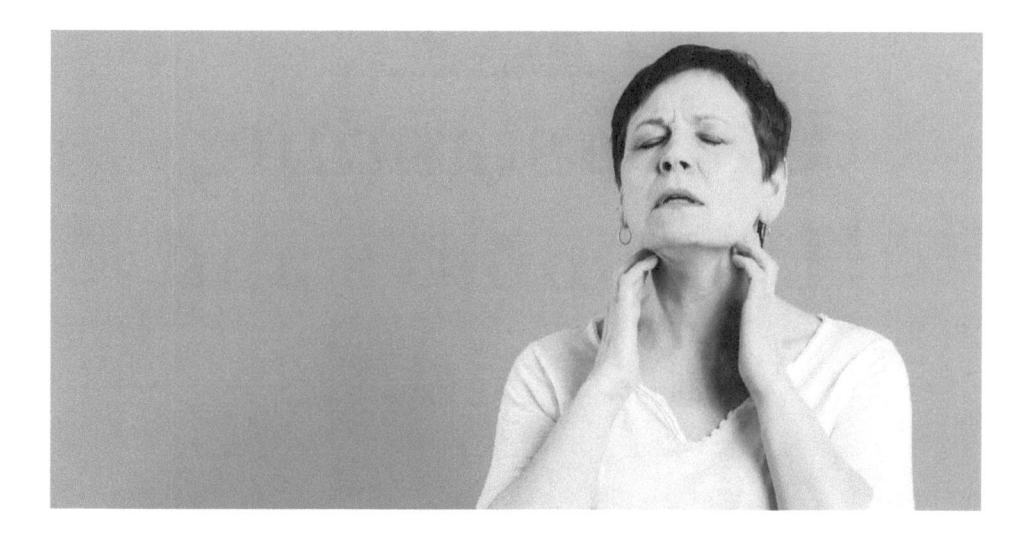

2.1: The Role of the Thyroid

The thyroid gland plays a pivotal role in regulating the body's metabolic processes. This butterfly-shaped organ, located at the base of your neck, is responsible for producing hormones that are critical for maintaining the body's metabolism. The hormones triiodothyronine (T3) and thyroxine (T4) are key players in controlling how your body uses energy, affecting nearly every organ in your body – from your heart and brain to your muscles and skin.

The significance of the thyroid extends beyond metabolism. It is instrumental in regulating body temperature, heart rate, and blood pressure. It also plays a vital role in supporting the body's growth and development and in the regulation of many bodily functions that contribute to overall health and well-being.

When the thyroid's function is compromised, as in Hashimoto's thyroiditis, the impact on the body can be profound. Hashimoto's thyroiditis leads to a decrease in the production of thyroid hormones, a condition known as hypothyroidism. This decline can cause a wide range of symptoms, including fatigue, weight gain, sensitivity to cold, constipation, dry skin, and hair loss. Over time, untreated hypothyroidism can lead to more serious health issues, such as heart problems, joint pain, and infertility.

The relationship between Hashimoto's thyroiditis and the immune system is also critical. In Hashimoto's, the immune system mistakenly attacks the thyroid gland, leading to inflammation and damage to the thyroid tissue. This autoimmune assault can alter the gland's ability to produce hormones, further exacerbating symptoms and complicating the condition.

Understanding the thyroid's role underscores the importance of managing Hashimoto's thyroiditis effectively. Strategies for managing this condition often include hormone replacement therapy to address the hormone deficiency caused by the damaged thyroid. However, managing Hashimoto's goes beyond just medication. It encompasses a holistic approach that includes dietary changes, stress management, and lifestyle adjustments to support thyroid health and mitigate the autoimmune response.

For those living with Hashimoto's, recognizing the signs and symptoms that indicate thyroid hormone levels may be off is crucial. Regular monitoring of thyroid function tests can help in adjusting treatment plans as needed. Additionally, adopting a diet rich in nutrients that support thyroid health, such as selenium, zinc, and iodine, and avoiding foods that can exacerbate inflammation, is beneficial.

Moreover, since stress can impact thyroid function and trigger or worsen autoimmune responses, incorporating stress-reduction techniques such as meditation, yoga, or deep-breathing exercises into daily routines can be advantageous. Regular physical activity is also essential, as it helps in weight management, improves energy levels, and contributes to overall well-being.

In essence, the thyroid gland's role in the body is multifaceted and critical for maintaining metabolic balance and overall health. For individuals with Hashimoto's thyroiditis, understanding this role is the first step towards effective management of the condition. Through a combination of medical treatment and lifestyle modifications, it is possible to manage the symptoms of Hashimoto's and lead a healthy, active life.

2.2: AUTOIMMUNITY IN HASHIMOTO'S EXPLAINED

At the core of Hashimoto's thyroiditis lies an **autoimmune response** where the body's immune system mistakenly targets the thyroid gland, leading to chronic inflammation and eventual deterioration of thyroid tissue. This autoimmune assault is not just an attack on the thyroid but a misdirected response of the immune system that can have far-reaching implications for the body's metabolic processes and overall health. The immune system, designed to protect the body against pathogens, turns against the thyroid gland, producing antibodies that attack the gland's cells. This ongoing battle results in the gradual destruction of thyroid tissue, impairing its ability to produce thyroid hormones, essential regulators of metabolism, energy, and body temperature.

The progression from a fully functioning thyroid to one that is underactive, a condition known as hypothyroidism, does not happen overnight. It is a slow, insidious process that can take years, during which the individual may experience a wide range of symptoms that can be mistakenly attributed to other causes. These symptoms include but are not limited to fatigue, weight gain, sensitivity to cold, dry skin, and constipation. The variability and commonality of these symptoms with other conditions often lead to misdiagnosis or delayed diagnosis, allowing the autoimmune process to continue unchecked.

The trigger for this autoimmune response is not fully understood but is believed to involve a combination of genetic predisposition and environmental factors. Certain genes increase susceptibility to autoimmune diseases, and when coupled with specific environmental triggers such as stress, infection, or exposure to certain chemicals, the risk of developing Hashimoto's increases. This complex interplay between genetics and environment highlights the multifaceted nature of the disease and the challenge in pinpointing a single cause.

Moreover, the immune system's attack on the thyroid gland leads to fluctuations in thyroid hormone levels, contributing to the complexity of managing Hashimoto's thyroiditis. The immune response can cause periods of inflammation that temporarily enhance hormone release, leading to transient symptoms of hyperthyroidism, such as anxiety, palpitations, and weight loss. However, as the disease progresses and more thyroid tissue is damaged, the predominant state becomes one of hypothyroidism.

The role of autoantibodies is central in the diagnosis and understanding of Hashimoto's. Thyroid peroxidase antibody (TPOAb) and thyroglobulin antibody (TgAb) are commonly elevated in individuals with Hashimoto's, serving as markers for the autoimmune process. The presence of these antibodies, along with characteristic symptoms and findings on thyroid function tests, helps in confirming the diagnosis.

Management of Hashimoto's thyroiditis focuses on alleviating symptoms and restoring normal thyroid hormone levels. Synthetic thyroid hormone replacement therapy is the mainstay of treatment, aiming to compensate for the underactive thyroid. However, addressing the autoimmune aspect of the disease requires a more holistic approach. Strategies such as optimizing nutrient intake, particularly selenium and vitamin D, which have been shown to reduce antibody levels, managing stress, and avoiding known dietary triggers, can help modulate the immune response and support thyroid health.

In conclusion, the journey of understanding and managing Hashimoto's thyroiditis involves recognizing the autoimmune nature of the disease, its gradual progression, and the complex interplay of factors that contribute to its development. By focusing on both the hormonal and autoimmune aspects of Hashimoto's, individuals can take proactive steps towards managing their symptoms and improving their quality of life.

2.3: COMMON SYMPTOMS AND MISDIAGNOSES

Individuals grappling with Hashimoto's thyroiditis often encounter a broad spectrum of symptoms that can mirror those of other conditions, leading to frequent misdiagnoses. The complexity of this autoimmune disorder lies in its ability to manifest through a variety of signs that are not unique to the thyroid gland's dysfunction. Recognizing these symptoms is crucial for accurate diagnosis and effective management.

Fatigue is one of the most prevalent symptoms, but it is also a common complaint in many other health issues, which makes it easy to overlook as a sign of thyroid dysfunction. The profound tiredness associated with Hashimoto's goes beyond the usual feelings of being tired after a long day; it's a deep, unrelenting fatigue that doesn't improve with rest.

Weight gain is another symptom that can be misinterpreted, as it is often attributed to poor diet, lack of exercise, or other metabolic disorders like Type 2 diabetes. However, in the context of Hashimoto's, weight gain occurs despite maintaining a healthy lifestyle, stemming from the slowed metabolism caused by decreased thyroid function.

Sensitivity to cold and feeling chilly in temperatures that others find comfortable can be dismissed as a personal quirk rather than a symptom of hypothyroidism. This sensitivity is due to the body's reduced ability to generate heat, a direct result of diminished thyroid hormone levels.

Constipation is a common gastrointestinal symptom that can be mistaken for dietary issues or irritable bowel syndrome. Yet, for those with Hashimoto's, constipation is a consequence of slowed bodily processes, including digestion, due to lower levels of thyroid hormones.

Dry skin and **hair loss** are often attributed to aging or skin conditions such as eczema. In individuals with Hashimoto's, these symptoms result from the slowed renewal of skin and hair cells, a process regulated by thyroid hormones.

Muscle weakness and **joint pain** can be misdiagnosed as arthritis, fibromyalgia, or simply attributed to aging. However, these symptoms in the context of Hashimoto's are often related to the inflammatory process of the autoimmune response and the overall decrease in metabolic function.

The **irregular menstrual periods** experienced by women with Hashimoto's can lead to diagnoses of polycystic ovary syndrome (PCOS) or other reproductive disorders. The disruption of menstrual cycles is directly linked to hormonal imbalances caused by thyroid dysfunction.

Given these symptoms' commonality with other conditions, it's not uncommon for individuals with Hashimoto's to be initially diagnosed with depression, chronic fatigue syndrome, or even anxiety disorders. The overlap of symptoms across these conditions can make it challenging for healthcare providers to recognize Hashimoto's without comprehensive thyroid function tests, including TSH, Free T4, Free T3, and thyroid antibody tests.

The key to differentiating Hashimoto's from other conditions lies in a careful evaluation of symptoms in conjunction with specific blood tests that can identify thyroid hormone levels and antibodies indicative of an autoimmune attack on the thyroid gland. It's essential for individuals experiencing these symptoms to advocate for thorough testing, especially if they have a family history of thyroid disorders or autoimmune diseases.

2.4: ROOT CAUSES OF THYROIDITIS: GUT, INFLAMMATION, STRESS

The intricate relationship between gut health, inflammation, and stress plays a pivotal role in the development and progression of thyroiditis, particularly in conditions such as Hashimoto's. The gut, often referred to as the "second brain," is home to a vast number of bacteria and immune cells that significantly influence the body's immune response. An imbalance in this gut microbiota, known as dysbiosis, can trigger an inflammatory response that extends beyond the gut, affecting distant organs, including the thyroid gland. This imbalance can stem from various factors, including diet, antibiotic use, and infections, leading to increased intestinal permeability, often dubbed "leaky gut." This condition allows substances that should be contained within the digestive tract to escape into the bloodstream, prompting an immune response that can contribute to or exacerbate autoimmune conditions like Hashimoto's.

Chronic inflammation is another critical factor in the development of thyroiditis. It can arise from persistent infections, obesity, poor diet, and autoimmune diseases. Inflammation in the body can disrupt the delicate balance of the immune system, leading to an increased production of antibodies against the body's own tissues, including the thyroid gland. This autoimmune attack results in the gradual destruction of thyroid cells, impairing hormone production and leading to the symptoms associated with Hashimoto's.

Stress, both physical and emotional, can significantly impact thyroid function. The body's stress response, mediated by the adrenal glands through the release of cortisol, can interfere with thyroid hormone production and utilization. Prolonged stress can lead to adrenal fatigue, which diminishes the body's ability to manage inflammation and can further impair immune function. Additionally, stress can exacerbate gut health issues, creating a vicious cycle that can initiate or worsen thyroid dysfunction.

To address these root causes, a multifaceted approach is necessary:

1. **Improving Gut Health**: Incorporating a diet rich in fiber, fermented foods, and nutrients that support the gut lining can help restore balance to the gut microbiota. Probiotics and prebiotics may also be beneficial in repopulating the gut with healthy bacteria.

2. **Reducing Inflammation**: Adopting an anti-inflammatory diet, rich in omega-3 fatty acids, antioxidants, and phytonutrients, can help reduce systemic inflammation. Regular physical activity and adequate sleep are also crucial in managing inflammatory responses.

3. **Managing Stress**: Techniques such as mindfulness meditation, yoga, and deep breathing exercises can be effective in reducing stress levels. Ensuring a healthy work-life balance and seeking support from friends, family, or professionals can also aid in stress management.

By addressing these underlying factors, individuals with Hashimoto's can take significant steps towards improving their condition. It is important to work closely with healthcare providers to develop a comprehensive plan that includes dietary changes, lifestyle modifications, and, when necessary, supplements or medications to support gut health, reduce inflammation, and manage stress.

symptoms but about creating a foundation for long-term health and well-being. Collaboration with healthcare providers to tailor a plan that considers unique health profiles and goals is crucial. Through targeted dietary changes, stress management techniques, and lifestyle adjustments, breaking free from the Hashimoto's vicious cycle becomes an achievable goal, paving the way for improved thyroid function, symptom relief, and enhanced quality of life.

3.2: BREAKING THE CYCLE: A NEW APPROACH TO HEALING

To effectively break the cycle of Hashimoto's, a holistic approach is necessary, focusing on diet, stress management, and hormonal balance. This strategy is not merely about symptom management but aims at addressing the root causes of the condition to foster long-term healing and well-being.

Dietary Adjustments: The foundation of disrupting the Hashimoto's cycle lies in dietary intervention. An anti-inflammatory diet plays a crucial role in this process. It involves eliminating foods that trigger inflammation, such as gluten, dairy, sugar, and processed foods, which are known to exacerbate autoimmune responses. Incorporating nutrient-dense foods that support thyroid health and reduce inflammation is essential. These include rich sources of selenium, such as Brazil nuts, and omega-3 fatty acids found in fatty fish like salmon. A focus on gut health is also paramount, with the inclusion of fermented foods like kefir and sauerkraut to replenish beneficial gut flora, alongside a high fiber intake from vegetables and fruits to support digestive health.

Stress Management Techniques: Chronic stress is a critical factor that can worsen Hashimoto's symptoms by affecting cortisol levels and, consequently, thyroid function. Implementing effective stress reduction techniques is vital. Practices such as mindfulness meditation, yoga, and tai chi can significantly lower stress levels. Additionally, engaging in regular physical activity not only reduces stress but also helps in managing weight and improving overall health. It's also beneficial to establish a routine that includes adequate sleep, as sleep deprivation can exacerbate both stress and inflammation, further impairing thyroid function.

Hormonal Balance Restoration: Hormonal imbalances play a significant role in the perpetuation of Hashimoto's thyroiditis. Managing these imbalances involves not only dietary and lifestyle changes but may also require supplementation and medication under the guidance of healthcare professionals. For example, optimizing vitamin D levels is crucial for immune function and hormonal health. Adaptogenic herbs, such as ashwagandha, have shown promise in supporting adrenal health and balancing cortisol levels, which can be particularly beneficial for those dealing with stress-induced exacerbation of Hashimoto's.

Environmental and Lifestyle Considerations: Minimizing exposure to environmental toxins by opting for organic produce, using natural cleaning products, and avoiding plastic containers can reduce the toxic burden on the body. Additionally, quitting smoking and limiting alcohol intake are critical steps in supporting overall health and reducing the risk factors associated with autoimmune diseases.

By integrating these strategies into daily life, individuals can take proactive steps towards breaking the cycle of Hashimoto's thyroiditis. It's a comprehensive approach that not only focuses on the physical aspects of healing but also acknowledges the importance of mental and emotional well-being in the healing process.

Chapter 4: Myths and Misconceptions About Hashimoto's

4.1: Debunking Myths About Diet, Medication, and Healing

Dispelling myths surrounding Hashimoto's thyroiditis is crucial for those on their healing journey. Misinformation can lead to confusion, frustration, and setbacks. This section aims to clarify some of the most pervasive myths about diet, medication, and the healing process, providing you with accurate information to support your path to better health.

Myth 1: A Specific Diet Can Cure Hashimoto's

While diet plays a significant role in managing Hashimoto's, no single diet can cure the condition. An anti-inflammatory diet can help reduce symptoms by lowering inflammation and supporting thyroid function. It's essential to find a dietary approach that works for you, focusing on whole foods and eliminating known triggers like gluten and dairy if they affect you negatively.

Myth 2: Medication Alone Is Enough to Manage Hashimoto's

Thyroid hormone replacement therapy, such as levothyroxine, is a standard treatment for Hashimoto's and can help manage symptoms by normalizing hormone levels. However, medication alone may not address all aspects of the condition. A comprehensive approach that includes diet, stress management, and lifestyle changes is often necessary for optimal health.

Myth 3: Supplements Can Replace Medication

While certain supplements can support thyroid health, such as selenium and vitamin D, they should not replace prescribed medications without a healthcare provider's guidance. Supplements can complement your treatment plan but should be used judiciously and in conjunction with other therapies.

Myth 4: Once Symptoms Improve, You Can Stop Focusing on Your Health

Hashimoto's is a lifelong condition, and while symptoms may improve with treatment, it doesn't mean the disease has disappeared. Continuing to maintain a healthy lifestyle, monitor your symptoms, and work with your healthcare provider is crucial for long-term management.

Myth 5: Hashimoto's Is Solely a Thyroid Problem

Hashimoto's is an autoimmune disease where the immune system attacks the thyroid. While it primarily affects the thyroid, it's a systemic issue that can influence other areas of the body. Addressing gut health, adrenal function, and systemic inflammation is essential for comprehensive management.

Myth 6: Everyone with Hashimoto's Will Experience the Same Symptoms

Symptoms of Hashimoto's can vary widely among individuals. While some may experience significant weight gain, fatigue, and cold intolerance, others may have mild symptoms or different manifestations of the condition. Tailoring treatment to the individual's symptoms and health status is crucial.

Myth 7: Iodine Supplements Are Beneficial for Everyone with Hashimoto's

Iodine plays a complex role in thyroid health. While it's essential for thyroid hormone production, excessive iodine can exacerbate Hashimoto's in some individuals. Before adding iodine supplements to your regimen, it's important to test your levels and consult with a healthcare provider.

Understanding these myths and the truths behind them empowers you to make informed decisions about your health. Collaborating with healthcare professionals who are knowledgeable about Hashimoto's can help you navigate the complexities of managing this condition, ensuring you adopt strategies that genuinely benefit your well-being.

4.2: THE TRUTH ABOUT LEVOTHYROXINE AND MEDICATIONS

Levothyroxine, a synthetic form of the thyroid hormone thyroxine (T4), plays a pivotal role in managing Hashimoto's thyroiditis by compensating for the underactive thyroid gland's reduced hormone production. This medication is crucial for normalizing metabolic functions and alleviating symptoms such as fatigue, weight gain, and cold sensitivity. Its effectiveness, however, is not solely dependent on the dosage but also on the consistency of its administration and the body's ability to absorb it. Factors that can affect levothyroxine absorption include gastrointestinal health, timing of ingestion relative to food and other medications, and the presence of certain supplements such as calcium and iron. To optimize the benefits of levothyroxine, it is recommended to take it on an empty stomach, ideally 30-60 minutes before breakfast or at bedtime, at least three hours after the last meal. This practice ensures maximum absorption and consistent thyroid hormone levels.

Other medications used in the management of Hashimoto's symptoms may include beta-blockers to control rapid heart rate and tremors in the initial phases of treatment, and selenium supplements, which some studies suggest could reduce thyroid antibody levels in people with Hashimoto's. However, it's important to consult with a healthcare provider before adding any supplements to your regimen, as their interaction with levothyroxine could alter its effectiveness.

Understanding the role of medication in managing Hashimoto's involves recognizing that while levothyroxine addresses the thyroid hormone deficiency, it does not halt the autoimmune attack on the thyroid gland. Comprehensive management of Hashimoto's may require addressing underlying autoimmune triggers, such as inflammation, dietary sensitivities, and stress, which can continue to affect thyroid function and overall health. Lifestyle modifications, including a nutrient-rich diet, stress reduction techniques, and regular exercise, complement the therapeutic effects of levothyroxine and other medications by supporting overall well-being and immune function.

Regular monitoring of thyroid function tests is essential to ensure that the dosage of levothyroxine remains optimal over time. As the thyroid gland's condition may change, and external factors such as weight, diet, and other health conditions evolve, adjustments to the medication dosage may be necessary to maintain thyroid hormone levels within the target range. Collaboration with an endocrinologist or a healthcare provider specializing in thyroid disorders is crucial for personalized medication management, allowing for adjustments based on symptoms, lab results, and individual response to treatment.

In the context of Hashimoto's thyroiditis, it's essential to view medications as part of a broader strategy that includes dietary interventions, lifestyle changes, and possibly other therapies aimed at reducing autoimmunity and supporting thyroid health. Patient education on the correct use of levothyroxine and open communication with healthcare providers about treatment goals and symptom management can significantly enhance quality of life for those living with Hashimoto's.

4.3: Symptom Management vs. Root Cause Healing

In the management of Hashimoto's thyroiditis, a clear distinction exists between **symptom management** and **root cause healing**. Symptom management involves addressing the immediate manifestations of the condition, such as fatigue, weight gain, and cold intolerance, often through medication and short-term dietary adjustments. While these approaches can provide relief, they do not necessarily address the underlying autoimmune process attacking the thyroid gland. In contrast, **root cause healing** aims to identify and address the foundational factors contributing to the autoimmune response, offering a more sustainable path to wellness.

Root cause healing focuses on several key areas:

1. **Gut Health:** A significant body of research links gut health with autoimmune conditions, including Hashimoto's. Addressing gut dysbiosis, healing intestinal permeability, and fostering a healthy microbiome can reduce systemic inflammation and autoimmune activity.

2. **Dietary Interventions:** Beyond eliminating symptomatic triggers like gluten or dairy, a deeper dietary approach focuses on reducing overall inflammation through nutrient-dense, whole foods. This strategy supports not only thyroid health but also immune regulation.

3. **Stress Management:** Chronic stress can exacerbate autoimmune activity by increasing cortisol levels and disrupting adrenal function. Techniques such as mindfulness, yoga, and adequate sleep are essential in mitigating stress's impact on the body.

4. **Toxin Exposure:** Reducing exposure to environmental toxins and addressing potential heavy metal accumulations in the body can decrease the burden on the immune system, lowering the risk of an autoimmune response.

5. **Nutritional Supplementation:** Targeted supplementation, including selenium, zinc, and vitamin D, can support thyroid function and immune balance, addressing specific deficiencies that may contribute to Hashimoto's.

6. **Lifestyle Modifications:** Regular physical activity, adequate hydration, and prioritizing sleep can profoundly impact overall health and resilience, supporting the body's natural healing processes.

By focusing on these areas, individuals can move beyond temporary symptom relief to achieve long-lasting health improvements. It's important to note that **root cause healing** is a personalized process; what works for one person may not work for another. Collaboration with healthcare providers knowledgeable in Hashimoto's and functional medicine can help tailor a healing plan to individual needs, incorporating both conventional and integrative approaches.

Embracing **root cause healing** requires patience, commitment, and a willingness to explore various aspects of health. While the path may be longer and more complex than symptom management alone, the potential for lasting wellness and a significantly improved quality of life makes it a worthwhile endeavor. Engaging actively in one's healing process, being open to adjustments in the plan, and maintaining a positive outlook are crucial components of success in addressing Hashimoto's at its roots.

Part 2:
Preparing for Success

Chapter 5: Preparing for Your 12-Week Plan

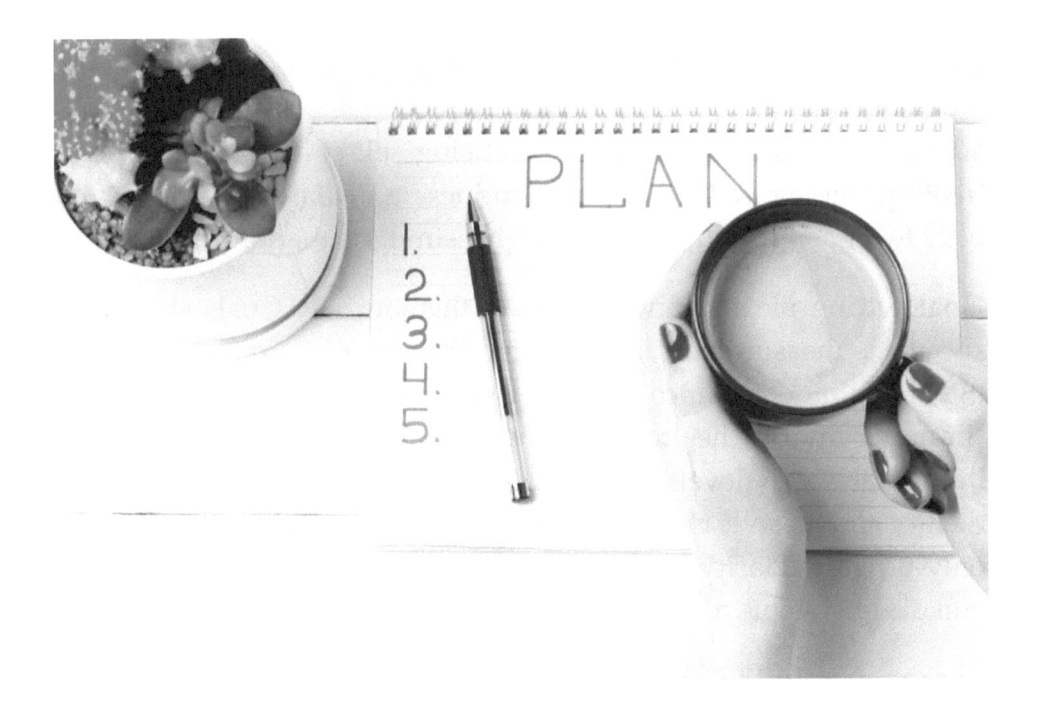

5.1: Setting Realistic Expectations

Embarking on a 12-week plan to address Hashimoto's thyroiditis requires a mindset geared towards gradual progress and patience. The first step in this process involves setting realistic expectations, which is fundamental to creating a sustainable path forward. It's important to understand that healing is not linear and each individual's response to the plan will vary based on numerous

Chapter 5:
Preparing for Your 12-Week Plan

factors including the severity of their condition, lifestyle, and adherence to the guidelines presented.

Realistic expectations should encompass an understanding that improvements in symptoms might not be immediate. The body needs time to adjust and respond to dietary changes, supplements, and lifestyle adjustments. It's also crucial to acknowledge that some weeks might yield more noticeable changes than others. This variability is completely normal and should not be a cause for discouragement.

Another key aspect is the **importance of self-compassion**. Healing from Hashimoto's is a journey that might include setbacks. These moments are not failures but opportunities for learning and adjusting the plan as needed. Practicing self-compassion involves treating oneself with the same kindness and patience one would offer to a good friend going through a similar situation.

Goal setting plays a pivotal role in this journey. Goals should be specific, measurable, achievable, relevant, and time-bound (SMART). For instance, rather than setting a vague goal like "improve thyroid health," a more targeted goal could be "reduce thyroid antibody levels by 20% within 12 weeks by adhering to the dietary and lifestyle changes outlined in the plan." This approach not only provides clarity but also makes it easier to track progress and make adjustments as needed.

Engagement in the process is equally important. This involves not just following the dietary and lifestyle recommendations but also actively participating in tracking symptoms, dietary intake, and any changes in how one feels. This active engagement helps in identifying patterns and correlations between certain activities or foods and symptoms, providing valuable insights that can guide further personalization of the plan.

Finally, **building a support system** can significantly enhance the healing journey. Whether it's family, friends, or online communities, having a network of individuals who understand and support your goals can provide encouragement and accountability. Additionally, regular consultations with healthcare providers not only help in monitoring progress but also in addressing any challenges that arise promptly.

In summary, setting realistic expectations is about understanding the nature of Hashimoto's healing process, practicing patience and self-compassion, setting clear and achievable goals, actively engaging in the healing process, and building a supportive network. These elements combined create a strong foundation for navigating the 12-week plan with resilience and optimism.

5.2 WORKBOOK EXERCISE: WRITING YOUR HEALTH VISION STATEMENT

> **Step 1:** Find a quiet, comfortable space where you can focus without interruptions. Have a notebook or a piece of paper and a pen ready.

> **Step 2:** Reflect on your current health status, focusing on how Hashimoto's has impacted your life. Think about your symptoms, energy levels, mood, weight, and overall well-being.

> **Step 3:** Visualize your optimal health scenario. Imagine a day in your life where Hashimoto's no longer controls your energy, mood, or diet. What does that look like? How do you feel waking up in the morning? What activities are you enjoying? How has your relationship with food changed?

> **Step 4:** Write down your health vision statement. Begin with "In my optimal health, I am..." and describe the vision you have for your health without Hashimoto's symptoms holding you back. Be as detailed and vivid as possible.

> Step 5: Consider the obstacles that might stand in the way of achieving this vision. Acknowledge these challenges but also write down strategies or resources that could help you overcome them.

> Step 6: Set small, achievable goals that will lead you towards your health vision. These could include dietary changes, incorporating specific supplements, daily movement, stress management techniques, or regular sleep schedules.

> Step 7: Create a commitment pledge to yourself. Write a statement that begins with "I commit to..." and list the actions you will take to achieve your health vision. Sign and date this pledge.

> Step 8: Share your health vision statement with a supportive friend, family member, or healthcare provider. Discussing your vision can provide additional motivation and accountability.

> Step 9: Revisit your health vision statement weekly. Update it as needed to reflect your journey, celebrating progress and reassessing goals to keep them aligned with your vision.

Chapter 6: Essential Tools for Healing

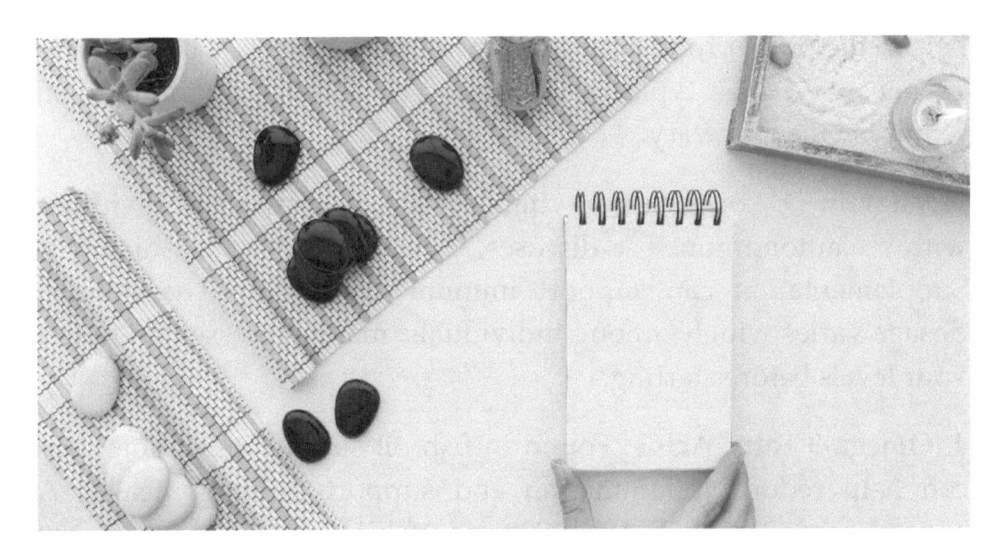

6.1: SUPPLEMENTS, LAB TESTS, AND RESOURCES

Embarking on the path to healing Hashimoto's thyroiditis requires a comprehensive approach that encompasses dietary changes, lifestyle adjustments, and the judicious use of supplements. Additionally, regular lab tests play a crucial role in monitoring your condition and the effectiveness of the interventions. Here, we'll delve into the essential supplements, lab tests, and resources you should consider at the outset of your healing journey.

Supplements

While no supplement can replace a balanced diet and proper medical care, certain nutrients have been shown to support thyroid health and immune function:

1. **Selenium**: This trace element is vital for the conversion of thyroid hormones from their inactive to active form. A daily dose of 200 mcg is often recommended, but it's crucial to consult with your healthcare provider to tailor the dosage to your needs.

2. **Zinc**: Zinc plays a significant role in hormone production and can help in the proper functioning of the immune system. A dosage of 8-11 mg per day is typically suggested for adults, but individual requirements may vary.

3. **Vitamin D**: Low levels of vitamin D are common in individuals with autoimmune diseases, including Hashimoto's. Supplementation can support immune regulation. The optimal dosage varies widely among individuals, making it essential to test your levels before starting.

4. **Omega-3 Fatty Acids**: Found in fish oil supplements, omega-3s can help reduce inflammation and support immune health. A general recommendation is 1,000 mg of EPA and DHA daily, but dosages should be personalized based on dietary intake and health status.

Lab Tests

Regular monitoring through lab tests is essential to assess the progression of Hashimoto's and the impact of any treatment strategy:

1. **Thyroid-Stimulating Hormone (TSH)**: This is the primary screening test for thyroid dysfunction, providing a snapshot of your thyroid's health.

2. **Free T4 and Free T3**: These tests measure the levels of active thyroid hormones in the bloodstream, offering insights into your metabolic rate.

3. **Thyroid Peroxidase Antibodies (TPOAb)** and **Thyroglobulin Antibodies (TgAb)**: Elevated levels of these antibodies indicate an autoimmune attack on the thyroid, a hallmark of Hashimoto's.

4. **Vitamin D**: Given its importance in immune function, testing for vitamin D levels can help guide supplementation.

5. **Complete Blood Count (CBC)** and **Comprehensive Metabolic Panel (CMP)**: These general health panels can provide clues about underlying issues that may affect thyroid health, such as inflammation or nutritional deficiencies.

Resources

To navigate your healing journey effectively, consider leveraging the following resources:

1. **Endocrinologists and Functional Medicine Practitioners**: Specialists who understand the intricacies of thyroid disorders can offer personalized care plans and support.

2. **Registered Dietitians**: Professionals specializing in autoimmune diseases can help design a diet that supports thyroid health and reduces inflammation.

3. **Support Groups**: Connecting with others facing similar challenges can provide emotional support, motivation, and practical advice.

4. **Educational Books and Websites**: Resources focusing on thyroid health, autoimmunity, and holistic healing can offer valuable insights and strategies.

5. **Health Tracking Apps**: Apps that track diet, supplements, and symptoms can help identify patterns and triggers, making it easier to adjust your approach as needed.

Chapter 6:
Essential Tools for Healing

Incorporating these supplements, undergoing regular lab tests, and utilizing available resources can empower you to take an active role in managing Hashimoto's thyroiditis. Remember, the most effective healing plan is personalized, taking into account your unique health situation, lifestyle, and goals. Collaboration with healthcare providers and a commitment to self-education and self-care are paramount in navigating the complexities of autoimmune thyroid disease.

6.2: Using Symptom Trackers and Food Journals

To effectively manage Hashimoto's thyroiditis, incorporating **symptom trackers and food journals** into your daily routine is invaluable. These tools not only provide insights into how different foods and lifestyle choices impact your well-being but also empower you to take control of your healing journey. Here's how to utilize these tools for optimal benefits:

Symptom Trackers: Keeping a detailed record of your symptoms on a daily basis allows you to notice patterns and triggers that may exacerbate your condition. This should include not only physical symptoms but also emotional well-being, energy levels, and sleep quality. Each entry should note the time of day and severity of the symptom on a scale, for example, from 1 to 10. Over time, this data can reveal correlations between your lifestyle choices and symptom fluctuations, guiding adjustments to your healing plan.

Food Journals: Documenting every meal, snack, and drink provides a comprehensive view of your nutritional intake and its effects on your health. Be sure to include portion sizes, ingredients, and any immediate reactions after eating, such as bloating, fatigue, or mood changes. This meticulous approach can help identify food sensitivities and intolerances, which are common in individuals with autoimmune conditions. Additionally, reviewing your food journal with a healthcare professional can offer further insights into nutritional deficiencies or dietary imbalances that need to be addressed.

Integrating Symptom Trackers and Food Journals: To maximize the utility of these tools, integrate your symptom tracking with your food journaling. This combined approach enables a holistic analysis of how diet directly correlates with symptom manifestation and severity. For instance, you may discover that consuming dairy products leads to increased joint pain or that sugar intake correlates with fatigue spikes. Armed with this knowledge, you can make informed decisions about dietary adjustments to alleviate your symptoms.

Review and Adjust: Regularly review your symptom tracker and food journal entries to assess progress and identify areas for improvement. This might be done weekly or bi-weekly, depending on your preference. Look for trends, such as improvements in symptoms following specific dietary changes or lifestyle adjustments. Use this information to continually refine your approach to managing Hashimoto's, whether that means tweaking your diet, altering your supplement regimen, or modifying your stress management techniques.

Digital Tools and Apps: Consider using digital platforms designed for health tracking to streamline this process. Many apps offer features for logging meals, symptoms, and lifestyle factors, along with analytics to easily visualize trends over time. Selecting an app that syncs with wearable devices can also provide additional data points, such as physical activity levels and sleep patterns, further enriching your insights.

Collaboration with Healthcare Providers: Share your findings from symptom tracking and food journaling with your healthcare team. This information can be invaluable during consultations, enabling more personalized and effective care. Your provider may offer suggestions based on your logs, such as eliminating certain foods or incorporating targeted supplements, to enhance your healing protocol.

By diligently using symptom trackers and food journals, you take an active role in your healing process, gaining the clarity and direction needed to navigate Hashimoto's thyroiditis with confidence. This practice not only fosters a deeper understanding of your body's responses but also equips you with the evidence-based insights necessary to optimize your health outcomes.

6.3 WORKBOOK EXERCISE: TRACKING YOUR CURRENT BASELINE (ENERGY, MOOD, SYMPTOMS)

Step 1: Gather a notebook or digital document dedicated to tracking your Hashimoto's healing journey. Label the first page as "Baseline Tracking."

Step 2: Divide the page into three sections: "Energy Levels," "Mood," and "Symptoms." Leave ample space under each section for detailed entries.

Step 3: Under "Energy Levels," rate your current energy level on a scale of 1 to 10, with 1 being extremely low energy and 10 being full of energy. Note the time of day when your energy feels highest and lowest.

Step 4: In the "Mood" section, describe your general mood and emotional state over the past week. Include any patterns you've noticed, such as times of day when you feel more anxious, depressed, or calm.

Step 5: List all current symptoms you are experiencing in the "Symptoms" section. Include as much detail as possible, like the severity of each symptom and how it impacts your daily life.

Step 6: For each section, write down any factors you believe are contributing to your current state. This could include diet, sleep quality, stress levels, and any other lifestyle factors.

Step 7: Set a reminder to review and update this baseline every week. Pay attention to any changes, no matter how small, and record them accordingly.

Step 8: Alongside this baseline tracking, start a daily journal entry noting your food intake, water consumption, physical activity, and any Hashimoto's medication or supplements you are taking. This will help you identify correlations between your lifestyle choices and your energy, mood, and symptoms over time.

Step 9: Share your baseline tracking with your healthcare provider at your next appointment. This can provide valuable insights for personalized care and adjustments to your healing plan.

Step 10: Reflect on your baseline tracking after the first month. Celebrate any improvements, no matter how minor, and consider adjustments for areas that haven't changed or have worsened. This ongoing process is crucial for understanding and managing your Hashimoto's effectively.

Part 3:
The 12-Week Healing Plan

Chapter 7: Reset and Detox

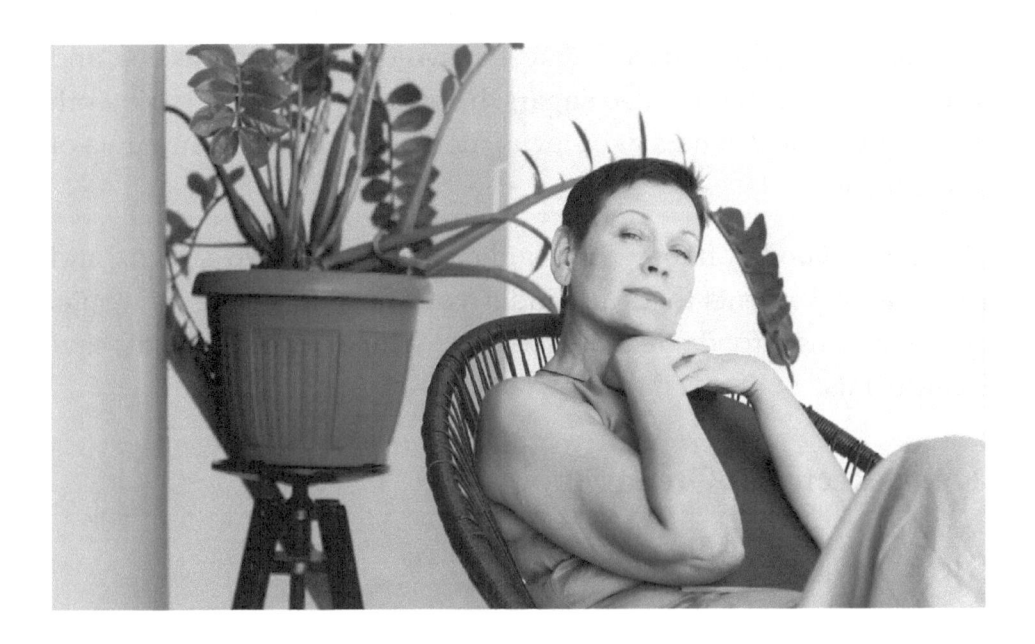

7.1: Eliminating Gluten, Dairy, Sugar, and Processed Foods

To initiate a healing process for Hashimoto's, identifying and eliminating common dietary triggers is crucial. Gluten, dairy, sugar, and processed foods are known to exacerbate inflammation and disrupt thyroid function. The following guide provides a structured approach to removing these items from your diet, along with three detox recipes to support your body's transition.

Gluten is a protein found in wheat, barley, and rye. Its inflammatory nature can lead to an immune response in individuals with Hashimoto's. Begin by replacing traditional bread, pasta, and baked goods with gluten-free alternatives made from rice, almond, or coconut flour.

Dairy products can also trigger inflammation due to lactose and casein. Opt for plant-based milk alternatives such as almond, coconut, or oat milk. Cheese and yogurt can be replaced with dairy-free versions made from nuts or soy.

Sugar contributes to inflammation, insulin resistance, and hormonal imbalances. Reduce your intake by avoiding sodas, sweets, and processed foods with added sugars. Instead, satisfy your sweet tooth with natural sweeteners like stevia, monk fruit, or small amounts of raw honey.

Processed Foods often contain unhealthy fats, added sugars, and artificial ingredients that can hinder your healing. Focus on whole, nutrient-dense foods like vegetables, fruits, lean proteins, and healthy fats.

Detox Recipe 1: Green Smoothie

- 1 cup spinach

- 1/2 avocado

- 1/2 cup pineapple chunks

- 1 tablespoon chia seeds

- 1 cup unsweetened almond milk

Blend all ingredients until smooth. This smoothie is rich in anti-inflammatory nutrients and healthy fats to support thyroid health.

Detox Recipe 2: Turmeric Ginger Tea

- 1 teaspoon turmeric

- 1/2 teaspoon grated ginger

- 1 tablespoon lemon juice

- 1 teaspoon raw honey (optional)

- 1 cup hot water

Combine turmeric, ginger, and hot water. Let steep for 5 minutes. Add lemon juice and honey to taste. Turmeric and ginger are powerful anti-inflammatory agents, while lemon boosts detoxification.

Detox Recipe 3: Quinoa Salad

- 1 cup cooked quinoa

- 1/2 cup diced cucumber

- 1/2 cup cherry tomatoes, halved

- 1/4 cup parsley, chopped

- 2 tablespoons olive oil

- 1 tablespoon apple cider vinegar

- Salt and pepper to taste

Mix all ingredients in a bowl. Quinoa provides a gluten-free source of protein and fiber, while vegetables add essential nutrients and fiber for detoxification.

Incorporating these dietary changes and recipes can significantly reduce inflammation and support your body's healing from Hashimoto's. Remember, the key to success is consistency and patience as your body adjusts to these healthier choices.

7.2: SUPPORTING LIVER HEALTH FOR DETOXIFICATION

The liver plays a crucial role in detoxifying the body, a process especially important for individuals managing Hashimoto's thyroiditis. To support liver health, incorporating specific foods and beverages that promote liver function and detoxification can make a significant difference in your healing journey. Here are practical recommendations for nourishing your liver, along with two detox beverage recipes and a list of beneficial supplements.

Foods that Support Liver Health:

- **Leafy Greens**: Spinach, kale, and collard greens are packed with chlorophyll, which assists the liver in removing toxins from the bloodstream.

- **Cruciferous Vegetables**: Broccoli, Brussels sprouts, and cauliflower increase the liver's ability to neutralize chemicals, hormones, and pesticides.

- **Garlic**: Rich in allicin and selenium, garlic activates liver enzymes that help flush out toxins.

- **Beets**: High in plant-flavonoids, beets improve overall liver function.

- **Green Tea**: Loaded with antioxidants, green tea supports the liver's detoxification processes.

- **Avocados**: They contribute to the production of glutathione, crucial for the liver's detoxification.

Detox Beverage Recipes:

1. **Liver Cleansing Beet Juice**:

   - 1 medium beet, peeled and chopped

   - 1 apple, cored and sliced

   - 1 carrot, peeled and chopped

   - ½ inch piece of fresh ginger

   - ½ lemon, peeled

   Juice all ingredients together for a powerful drink that not only supports liver health but also boosts your intake of essential vitamins and minerals.

2. **Refreshing Turmeric Liver Detox Tea**:

   - 1 teaspoon turmeric powder

   - 1 teaspoon grated ginger

   - Juice of ½ lemon

   - 1 tablespoon raw honey

   - 1 cup hot water

   Combine turmeric, ginger, and hot water in a mug. Allow to steep for 10 minutes, then add lemon juice and honey. This tea is not only soothing but packed with anti-inflammatory properties that support liver function.

Supplements for Liver Health:

- **Milk Thistle**: Known for its protective effects on the liver, milk thistle supports liver cell regeneration and detoxification.

- **Dandelion Root**: Traditionally used to support liver health, dandelion root stimulates bile flow and helps purify the liver and gallbladder.

- **Turmeric**: This spice supports the liver's detoxification processes, thanks to its potent antioxidant properties.

- **Omega-3 Fatty Acids**: Found in fish oil, these fatty acids reduce inflammation and support liver health.

- **N-acetylcysteine (NAC)**: Helps replenish glutathione levels, a critical antioxidant for detoxification processes in the liver.

Incorporating these foods, beverages, and supplements into your daily routine can significantly support your liver's health, enhancing your body's detoxification processes and contributing to your overall well-being as you navigate the path to healing Hashimoto's thyroiditis. Remember, always consult with your healthcare provider before adding any new supplements to your regimen to ensure they align with your specific health needs and conditions.

7.3 WORKBOOK EXERCISE: DAILY FOOD TRACKER AND DETOX CHECKLIST

Step 1: Prepare your Daily Food Tracker and Detox Checklist. Use a digital app or a physical notebook, whichever suits your preference. Label the top of the page with today's date.

Step 2: Divide the tracker into four sections: "Meals," "Water Intake," "Symptoms," and "Detox Activities."

Step 3: Under "Meals," record everything you eat and drink throughout the day. Include portion sizes and the time of each meal or snack. Be as detailed as possible to notice patterns later.

Step 4: In the "Water Intake" section, keep track of how many ounces of water you drink. Aim for at least 64 ounces (about 1.9 liters) daily to support detoxification and hydration.

Step 5: Use the "Symptoms" section to note any physical or emotional symptoms you experience during the day. Include the time symptoms occur and rate their severity on a scale of 1 to 10.

Step 6: The "Detox Activities" section is for tracking any specific detox-related actions you take, such as consuming detox teas, taking liver-support supplements, engaging in light exercise, or practicing stress-reduction techniques like meditation or deep breathing.

Step 7: At the end of the day, review your Daily Food Tracker and Detox Checklist. Reflect on any correlations between your diet, detox activities, and symptoms. Consider what changes, if any, could be beneficial for the following day.

Step 8: Set a goal for the next day based on your reflections. This could involve increasing water intake, adjusting portion sizes, adding or removing certain foods, or incorporating more detox activities into your routine.

Step 9: Repeat this process daily throughout the first two weeks of your Reset and Detox phase. Consistent tracking will help you identify what works best for your body and can lead to more informed decisions about your health moving forward.

Step 10: Share insights from your tracker with your healthcare provider, especially if you notice persistent symptoms or have concerns about your detox plan. This can help tailor the plan to your specific needs for optimal healing.

Chapter 8:
Rebuild and Nourish

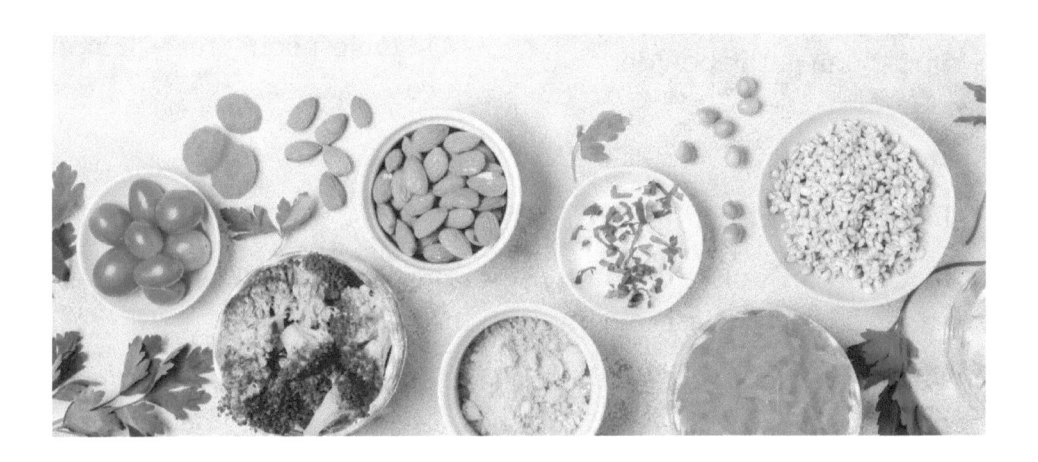

8.1: INCORPORATING ANTI-INFLAMMATORY FOODS

Inflammation plays a pivotal role in the exacerbation of Hashimoto's thyroiditis, making the incorporation of anti-inflammatory foods into one's diet an essential strategy for managing this condition. These foods work by reducing the body's inflammatory responses, thus potentially mitigating the autoimmune attack on the thyroid gland. Below are three nutrient-rich recipes designed to nourish your body and combat inflammation.

Turmeric Chicken & Vegetables

Ingredients:

- 2 boneless, skinless chicken breasts
- 1 tablespoon olive oil
- 1 teaspoon ground turmeric
- ½ teaspoon garlic powder
- Salt and pepper to taste
- 2 cups mixed vegetables (broccoli, bell peppers, and carrots)
- 1 tablespoon fresh lemon juice

Instructions:

1. Preheat your oven to 375°F (190°C).

2. In a bowl, mix olive oil, turmeric, garlic powder, salt, and pepper. Coat the chicken breasts evenly with the mixture.

3. Place the chicken on a baking sheet. Surround it with the mixed vegetables.

4. Bake for 25-30 minutes, until the chicken is thoroughly cooked and the vegetables are tender.

5. Drizzle lemon juice over the chicken and vegetables before serving. This dish combines the powerful anti-inflammatory properties of turmeric with the nutrient density of fresh vegetables, creating a balanced meal that supports thyroid health.

Salmon with Avocado Salsa

Ingredients:

- 2 salmon fillets
- 1 ripe avocado, diced
- 1 small red onion, finely chopped
- 1 tomato, diced
- Juice of 1 lime
- 2 tablespoons chopped cilantro
- Salt and pepper to taste
- 1 tablespoon olive oil

Instructions:

1. Preheat the grill to medium-high heat.

2. Season the salmon fillets with salt and pepper, then brush them with olive oil.

3. Grill the salmon for about 5 minutes on each side, or until cooked to your liking.

4. In a bowl, mix the avocado, red onion, tomato, lime juice, cilantro, salt, and pepper to create the salsa.

5. Serve the grilled salmon topped with the fresh avocado salsa. The omega-3 fatty acids in salmon reduce inflammation, while avocado provides healthy fats that promote hormone balance and support thyroid function.

Spinach and Berry Smoothie

Ingredients:

- 1 cup fresh spinach
- ½ cup mixed berries (blueberries, strawberries, raspberries)
- 1 banana
- 1 tablespoon chia seeds
- 1 cup almond milk
- A handful of ice cubes

Instructions:

1. Place all ingredients in a blender.

2. Blend on high until smooth and creamy.

3. Serve immediately. This smoothie is not only refreshing but packed with antioxidants from the berries and spinach, fiber from the banana, and omega-3s from the chia seeds, all of which are known to have anti-inflammatory effects.

By integrating these recipes into your weekly meal plan, you can enjoy delicious and healthful meals that contribute to reducing inflammation and supporting your thyroid health. Remember, the key to managing Hashimoto's effectively lies in consistent dietary choices that focus on whole, unprocessed foods rich in nutrients that combat inflammation and support overall well-being.

8.2: Key Nutrients for Thyroid Function

For optimal thyroid function, ensuring adequate intake of **selenium**, **zinc**, and **vitamin D** is crucial. Each of these nutrients plays a vital role in supporting thyroid health and overall well-being. Here, we provide detailed information on the importance of these nutrients, along with two recipes for each to help incorporate them into your diet effortlessly.

Selenium is essential for the conversion of thyroid hormones from T4 to the more active form, T3. It also protects the thyroid gland from oxidative damage due to its antioxidant properties. Foods rich in selenium include Brazil nuts, seafood, and mushrooms.

Recipe 1: Brazil Nut Smoothie

- 2 Brazil nuts
- 1 cup almond milk
- 1 banana
- 1 tablespoon chia seeds
- 1 cup spinach

Blend all ingredients until smooth. This smoothie is not only a powerhouse of selenium but also provides fiber and healthy fats.

Recipe 2: Seared Scallops with Mushroom Sauce

- 4 large scallops
- 1 tablespoon olive oil
- 1 cup sliced mushrooms
- Salt and pepper to taste
- 1 garlic clove, minced

Sear scallops in olive oil over medium-high heat until golden brown. Saute mushrooms and garlic in the same pan, adding a splash of water to deglaze. Serve scallops topped with mushroom sauce. This dish is an excellent way to boost your selenium intake.

Zinc is crucial for thyroid hormone synthesis and metabolism. It also aids in immune system support, which is vital for individuals with Hashimoto's. High-zinc foods include beef, pumpkin seeds, and lentils.

Recipe 1: Pumpkin Seed Pesto

- 1 cup fresh basil leaves
- 1/2 cup pumpkin seeds, toasted
- 1/2 cup grated Parmesan cheese
- 1/2 cup olive oil
- 2 garlic cloves, minced

Combine all ingredients in a food processor until smooth. This pesto is versatile and can be used with pasta, as a spread, or a dip, providing a delicious way to add zinc to your diet.

Recipe 2: Beef and Lentil Stew

- 1 pound lean beef, cubed
- 1 cup lentils
- 1 onion, chopped
- 2 carrots, chopped
- 4 cups beef broth
- Salt and pepper to taste

Cook all ingredients in a slow cooker on low for 8 hours. This hearty stew is not only comforting but also rich in zinc, supporting thyroid and immune health.

Vitamin D is not only essential for bone health but also plays a significant role in modulating the immune system and reducing inflammation. While sunlight is a primary source, foods like fatty fish, egg yolks, and fortified foods can also contribute to vitamin D intake.

Recipe 1: Salmon with Lemon and Dill

- 2 salmon fillets
- Juice of 1 lemon
- 1 tablespoon fresh dill, chopped
- Salt and pepper to taste

Bake salmon at 375°F (190°C) for 20 minutes, topped with lemon juice, dill, salt, and pepper. This simple yet flavorful dish is an excellent source of vitamin D.

Recipe 2: Spinach and Mushroom Omelet

- 2 eggs
- 1 cup spinach
- 1/2 cup sliced mushrooms
- 1/4 cup shredded cheese
- Salt and pepper to taste

Saute spinach and mushrooms, then add beaten eggs and cheese, cooking until the eggs are set. This omelet is a tasty way to start your day with a boost of vitamin D.

Incorporating these nutrients into your daily meals can significantly support thyroid health and overall vitality. Remember, while diet plays a crucial role in managing Hashimoto's, it's essential to consult with a healthcare provider to tailor a plan that meets your specific needs.

8.3 WORKBOOK EXERCISE: WEEKLY MEAL PLANNING

Step 1: Choose a day to plan your weekly meals, ideally a few days before your grocery shopping day. This allows time to make any necessary adjustments to your plan.

Step 2: Create a meal planning template or use a digital app. Your template should have sections for each day of the week and slots for breakfast, lunch, dinner, and snacks.

Step 3: Review the key nutrients for thyroid function from Chapter 8.2, focusing on incorporating foods rich in selenium, zinc, and vitamin D into your meals. Examples include Brazil nuts for selenium, pumpkin seeds for zinc, and fatty fish like salmon for vitamin D.

Step 4: Draft your meal plan, aiming for variety and balance. Start with dinners, as they typically require more preparation, and then plan your lunches, breakfasts, and snacks. Consider how dinner leftovers can serve as next day's lunch to save time and reduce waste.

Step 5: Write down your meal plan, including specific dishes for each meal slot. For example:

- Monday Dinner: Baked Salmon with Asparagus (rich in vitamin D and selenium)

- Tuesday Lunch: Leftover Salmon Salad

Step 6: After planning your meals, create a shopping list organized by grocery store sections (produce, meat, dairy, etc.). This will streamline your shopping process and help ensure you don't forget any ingredients.

Step 7: Check your pantry and fridge to cross off items you already have before heading to the grocery store. This prevents duplicate purchases and helps manage your food budget.

Step 8: Incorporate one new recipe each week to gradually expand your dietary variety. This could be a new way to prepare a familiar vegetable or a dish from a different cuisine that includes the recommended nutrients.

Step 9: Prepare any components of your meals that can be made in advance. For example, chopping vegetables, cooking quinoa, or making a batch of homemade dressing can save time during the week.

Step 10: Reflect at the end of the week on what meals worked well and which ones didn't. Adjust your plan for the next week based on what you learned. Did you find certain meals kept you more satisfied or energized? Were there recipes that were too time-consuming for your schedule?

Step 11: Remember to stay flexible. Life can be unpredictable, so if you need to swap meals around or substitute ingredients based on what's available, that's perfectly fine. The goal is to nourish your body while supporting your thyroid health, not to follow the plan perfectly.

Chapter 9: Gut Health and Hormonal Balance

9.1: HEALING THE GUT WITH PROBIOTICS AND ENZYMES

The gut plays a pivotal role in overall health, particularly for those battling Hashimoto's thyroiditis. A balanced intestinal flora and efficient digestion are crucial in reducing autoimmunity and promoting hormonal balance. Incorporating probiotics and enzymes into your diet can significantly enhance gut health, aiding in the absorption of nutrients and the reduction of inflammation. Here are three recipes to help support your intestinal health with beneficial probiotics and digestive enzymes.

Fermented Carrot and Ginger Salad

Ingredients:

- 5 large carrots, peeled and thinly sliced
- 2 tablespoons grated fresh ginger
- 1 clove garlic, minced
- 2 teaspoons sea salt
- 4 tablespoons whey or a probiotic capsule (if dairy-free)

Instructions:

1. In a large bowl, combine the carrots, ginger, and garlic. Sprinkle with sea salt and massage the mixture with your hands for about 5 minutes, until there is a noticeable release of liquid.

2. Stir in the whey or open the probiotic capsule and mix thoroughly.

3. Pack the mixture into a clean, quart-sized glass jar, leaving at least 1 inch of space at the top. Press down firmly until the liquid rises above the solids.

4. Cover the jar with a tight lid and let it sit at room temperature for 3-5 days. Check daily to ensure the vegetables are submerged, pressing down if necessary.

5. Once fermented, store in the refrigerator. The salad can be enjoyed as a flavorful side dish, providing a rich source of probiotics to support gut health.

Pineapple Papaya Smoothie

Ingredients:

- 1 cup fresh pineapple, diced
- 1 cup fresh papaya, diced
- 1 banana
- 1 cup coconut water or almond milk
- 1 tablespoon honey (optional)
- A pinch of ground cinnamon

Instructions:

1. Combine all ingredients in a blender.

2. Blend until smooth. If the mixture is too thick, add a little more coconut water or almond milk to reach the desired consistency.

3. Enjoy immediately. This smoothie is not only refreshing but also packed with natural enzymes from pineapple and papaya, aiding in digestion and nutrient absorption.

Kefir Overnight Oats

Ingredients:

- ½ cup rolled oats
- 1 cup kefir
- 1 tablespoon chia seeds
- 1 tablespoon maple syrup or honey
- ½ teaspoon vanilla extract
- Toppings: fresh berries, nuts, seeds, or coconut flakes

Instructions:

1. In a mason jar or bowl, combine the oats, kefir, chia seeds, maple syrup, and vanilla extract. Stir well.

2. Cover and refrigerate overnight.

3. In the morning, stir the oats and add a little more kefir if needed to adjust the consistency.

4. Top with fresh berries, nuts, seeds, or coconut flakes before serving. This breakfast option is an excellent way to start your day with a dose of probiotics from kefir, along with fiber from oats and chia seeds, promoting a healthy digestive system.

By integrating these recipes into your diet, you can support your gut health, which is essential for managing Hashimoto's thyroiditis. Remember, a healthy gut contributes to a strong immune system, improved digestion, and a balanced hormonal environment, all of which are vital for your healing journey.

9.2: REDUCING CORTISOL AND SUPPORTING ADRENAL HEALTH

High levels of cortisol, often referred to as the "stress hormone," can wreak havoc on your body, particularly for those managing Hashimoto's thyroiditis. Elevated cortisol can lead to hormonal imbalances, disrupt your metabolism, and exacerbate thyroid issues. Fortunately, certain foods have properties that can help lower cortisol levels and support adrenal health, which is crucial for rebalancing hormones and promoting overall well-being. Below are two recipes designed to nourish your body and help mitigate stress on a physiological level.

Ashwagandha Moon Milk

Ashwagandha, an adaptogenic herb, has been shown to significantly reduce cortisol levels, making it an excellent addition to your diet for stress management.

Ingredients:

- 1 cup almond milk
- ½ teaspoon ashwagandha powder
- 1 tsp honey or maple syrup
- ¼ teaspoon cinnamon
- A pinch of nutmeg and cardamom

Instructions:

1. Gently heat the almond milk in a small saucepan over low heat until it is just warm.

2. Whisk in the ashwagandha powder, ensuring there are no clumps.

3. Stir in the honey or maple syrup, cinnamon, nutmeg, and cardamom.

4. Pour into a mug and enjoy before bedtime to promote relaxation and a restful night's sleep.

Salmon Avocado Salad

Omega-3 fatty acids, found abundantly in salmon, have been proven to reduce cortisol levels and inflammation. Avocado adds a healthy dose of monounsaturated fats, which are beneficial for hormonal balance.

Ingredients:

- 2 salmon fillets, grilled and flaked
- 1 ripe avocado, diced
- 2 cups mixed greens (spinach, arugula, and kale)
- ½ cucumber, sliced
- ¼ cup red onion, thinly sliced
- 2 tablespoons olive oil
- Juice of 1 lemon
- Salt and pepper to taste
- A handful of walnuts for garnish

Instructions:

1. In a large bowl, combine the mixed greens, cucumber, and red onion.

2. Add the grilled, flaked salmon and diced avocado to the bowl.

3. In a small bowl, whisk together the olive oil, lemon juice, salt, and pepper to create a dressing.

4. Pour the dressing over the salad and toss gently to coat evenly.

5. Garnish with walnuts before serving. This salad is not only delicious but also packed with nutrients that support adrenal health and help lower cortisol levels.

Incorporating these recipes into your diet can be a step towards managing stress and supporting your body's hormonal balance. Remember, diet is just one component of a holistic approach to healing Hashimoto's thyroiditis. Regular exercise, adequate sleep, and stress-reduction techniques like meditation and yoga are also crucial for lowering cortisol levels and enhancing your overall health.

9.3 WORKBOOK EXERCISE: TRACKING DIGESTIVE CHANGES

Step 1: Obtain a dedicated journal or digital document for tracking digestive changes. Title the first section "Digestive Health Baseline."

Step 2: Record your current digestive symptoms, including bloating, gas, constipation, diarrhea, or any discomfort. Rate each symptom on a scale from 1 to 10, with 1 being mild and 10 being severe.

Step 3: Note any foods you suspect may be contributing to your symptoms. Include the time of day these foods were consumed and any immediate reactions you observed.

Step 4: Start incorporating the recommended anti-inflammatory foods and probiotics into your diet. List these foods in your journal along with the date of incorporation.

Step 5: Each day, track your consumption of these foods and any changes in your digestive symptoms. Be specific about the time of day and the quantities consumed.

Step 6: Monitor your water intake, aiming for at least 64 ounces (about 1.9 liters) per day. Record the amount of water you drink daily in your journal.

Step 7: Pay attention to your stress levels and their impact on your digestive health. Briefly document any stress-reducing activities you engage in, such as meditation, yoga, or deep breathing exercises.

Step 8: Weekly, summarize your observations, noting any patterns or correlations between dietary changes, stress management, and symptom improvement or worsening.

Step 9: After 2 weeks, review your notes to identify which changes have been most effective in improving your symptoms. Adjust your diet and lifestyle practices based on these insights.

Step 10: Continue this tracking and adjusting process throughout the 12-week plan, always aiming to refine your approach to support optimal gut health and hormonal balance.

Step 11: Share your findings and progress with your healthcare provider to tailor any medical advice or interventions to your specific needs and responses.

Chapter 10: Energy Restoration in Weeks 7-8

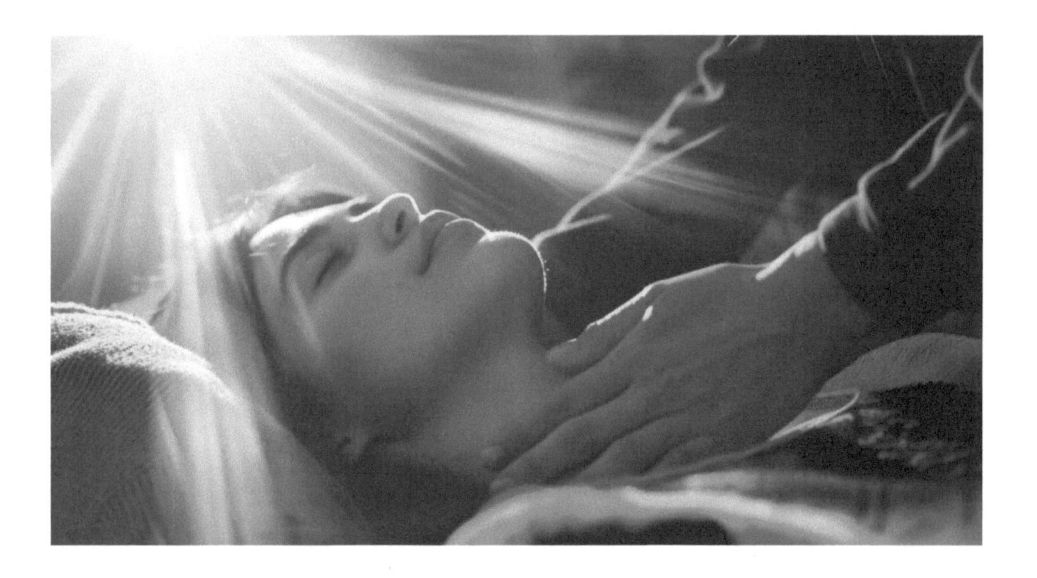

10.1: COMBATING FATIGUE WITH SLEEP, MOVEMENT, AND HYDRATION

Chronic fatigue can be a significant obstacle for individuals managing Hashimoto's, but addressing sleep, incorporating movement, and focusing on hydration can be transformative. Establishing a restorative sleep routine is paramount. Aim for 7-9 hours of quality sleep each night. Create a calming bedtime ritual and maintain a consistent sleep schedule, even on weekends. The goal is to support your body's natural circadian rhythms, which can, in turn, help regulate thyroid function.

Hydration plays a crucial role in energy levels. Dehydration can exacerbate fatigue, making it essential to drink at least 8-10 glasses of water daily. Consider starting your day with a glass of lemon water to kickstart digestion and hydration. Throughout the day, herbal teas and infused waters with cucumber, mint, or berries can add variety and support hydration.

Movement is equally vital. Incorporate gentle, restorative exercises such as walking, yoga, or tai chi. These activities can boost energy without overtaxing the body. Aim for at least 30 minutes of moderate exercise most days of the week, but listen to your body and adjust as needed. Movement not only improves circulation and energy but also supports mood and hormone balance.

To complement these strategies, here are **three energizing breakfast recipes** that are easy to prepare and thyroid-friendly:

1. Berry Chia Seed Pudding

- 3 tablespoons of chia seeds
- 1 cup of unsweetened almond milk
- ½ teaspoon of vanilla extract
- 1 tablespoon of maple syrup or honey (optional)
- ½ cup of mixed berries
- A sprinkle of cinnamon (optional)

Mix the chia seeds, almond milk, vanilla, and sweetener in a bowl. Let it sit overnight in the refrigerator. In the morning, top with fresh berries and a sprinkle of cinnamon for an added flavor boost. This breakfast is rich in omega-3 fatty acids and fiber, promoting satiety and supporting gut health.

2. Spinach and Mushroom Omelette

- 2 eggs
- 1 cup of fresh spinach
- ½ cup of sliced mushrooms
- 1 tablespoon of olive oil
- Salt and pepper to taste
- A sprinkle of turmeric (optional for anti-inflammatory benefits)

Heat the olive oil in a skillet, sauté the mushrooms until golden, then add the spinach until wilted. Beat the eggs with salt, pepper, and turmeric, then pour over the veggies in the skillet. Cook until the eggs are set and enjoy. This protein-rich meal supports sustained energy levels and thyroid health.

3. Quinoa Breakfast Bowl

- ½ cup of cooked quinoa
- 1 tablespoon of flaxseed
- 1 apple, diced
- A handful of walnuts
- A dash of cinnamon
- Unsweetened almond milk to serve

Combine the cooked quinoa, flaxseed, diced apple, and walnuts in a bowl. Add a dash of cinnamon for flavor and pour almond milk over the mixture. This breakfast bowl is high in protein, fiber, and essential fatty acids, all of which support energy levels and thyroid health.

Incorporating these strategies and recipes into your daily routine can significantly impact your energy levels, helping to combat chronic fatigue associated with Hashimoto's. Remember, small, consistent changes can lead to substantial improvements in your overall well-being.

10.2 WORKBOOK EXERCISE: ENERGY TRACKER AND SELF-CARE PLANNER

Step 1: Obtain a notebook or digital app specifically for your Energy Tracker and Self-Care Planner. This will be your dedicated space to monitor and plan your daily energy levels and self-care activities.

Step 2: At the beginning of each day, rate your initial energy level on a scale from 1 to 10, with 1 being extremely low energy and 10 being full of energy. Record this rating in your tracker.

Step 3: Below your morning energy rating, jot down any specific goals or intentions for self-care that day. This could include activities such as a 20-minute walk, meditation, reading for pleasure, or taking a relaxing bath.

Step 4: Throughout the day, keep a log of your meals, hydration, and any snacks. Note the times you eat and drink, as maintaining a balanced diet and staying hydrated can significantly impact your energy levels.

Step 5: Track your physical activity, including the type of activity, duration, and how you felt afterward. Physical movement can boost energy, so finding a balance that works for you is key.

Step 6: Monitor your sleep from the night before, including how many hours you slept and the quality of your sleep. Good sleep hygiene is crucial for energy restoration.

Step 7: At the end of the day, rate your energy level again on a scale from 1 to 10. Reflect on any fluctuations throughout the day and what activities or meals may have contributed to these changes.

Step 8: Review the self-care activities you had planned for the day. Did you accomplish them? If not, what barriers did you encounter? Use this reflection to adjust your plans for the next day, keeping in mind realistic and achievable goals.

Step 9: Weekly, take some time to review your energy and self-care logs. Look for patterns or trends that emerge. Are there certain foods, activities, or sleep patterns that consistently seem to affect your energy levels?

Step 10: Based on your weekly review, set specific goals for the following week. These could include trying a new type of physical activity, adjusting your bedtime routine, or incorporating more of a certain nutrient into your diet.

Step 11: Remember, this is a personal and flexible tool designed to help you understand and improve your energy levels and overall well-being. Adjust the tracking and planning process as needed to fit your lifestyle and health goals.

Chapter 11: Long-Term Maintenance

11.1: Reintroducing Foods and Monitoring Reactions

After weeks of following a strict elimination diet to manage Hashimoto's, the reintroduction phase is a critical step towards understanding your body's responses to different foods. This process involves systematically reintroducing foods that were previously eliminated, one at a time, to monitor for any adverse reactions. These reactions can provide valuable insights into which foods your body can tolerate and which may be contributing to your symptoms. The goal is to create a personalized diet that supports your thyroid health while maximizing nutritional intake.

Step 1: Choose the Right Time

Begin reintroducing foods when you are feeling relatively symptom-free and are not experiencing significant stress. This stable period makes it easier to discern any changes that occur as a result of reintroducing a specific food.

Step 2: Select a Food to Reintroduce

Start with foods that are less likely to cause a reaction, such as those with low allergenic potential. Common examples include fermented dairy products like kefir or yogurt, eggs, and legumes. Keep a detailed food diary during this phase to note what you're reintroducing and any symptoms you experience.

Step 3: Introduce One Food at a Time

Introduce one single food over a period of 3-4 days, starting with a small amount on the first day and gradually increasing it if no reaction occurs. For instance, if reintroducing eggs, you might start with eating a quarter of an egg and observe any symptoms for at least three days.

Step 4: Monitor Symptoms

Pay close attention to any changes in your symptoms, including digestive upset, fatigue, skin reactions, or any other Hashimoto's symptoms. Use a symptom tracker to record your observations, noting the type and severity of any reactions.

Step 5: Evaluate the Results

If no adverse reactions are observed after 3-4 days, you can consider the food as tolerated and incorporate it into your diet. However, if you experience negative symptoms, remove the food from your diet again and allow your body to recover before attempting to reintroduce another food.

Step 6: Repeat the Process

Continue this process, one food at a time, until you have tested all the foods you wish to reintroduce. This meticulous approach helps to identify specific foods that you may need to avoid to manage your Hashimoto's effectively.

Additional Tips for Success

- Keep a detailed journal throughout this process to record not only the foods you reintroduce and the symptoms you experience but also any other relevant factors such as stress levels, sleep quality, and exercise. This comprehensive view can help you identify patterns and triggers more accurately.

- Consider working with a healthcare professional, such as a dietitian or a functional medicine doctor, who can provide guidance tailored to your specific needs and help interpret your reactions.

- Listen to your body and proceed at a pace that feels comfortable for you. There's no rush in this phase, and taking the time to understand your body's responses can provide invaluable insights for long-term management of Hashimoto's.

By carefully following these steps, you can develop a diet that supports your health and wellbeing, taking into account your body's unique responses to different foods. This personalized approach is key to managing Hashimoto's effectively and improving your quality of life.

11.2: BUILDING RESILIENCE AGAINST RELAPSES

Building resilience against relapses in Hashimoto's management involves a strategic approach to nutrition and lifestyle that prioritizes sustainability and balance. This focus ensures that the body receives consistent support to maintain thyroid health and overall well-being. To facilitate this, incorporating meals that are not only nutritious but also easy to prepare and integrate into a busy lifestyle is essential. These recipes are designed to provide balanced nutrition, support thyroid function, and prevent relapses by keeping inflammation and autoimmune triggers at bay.

Chapter 11:
Long-Term Maintenance

Sustainable Salmon Quinoa Salad

Ingredients:

- 4 ounces of wild-caught salmon

- 1/2 cup of cooked quinoa

- 1 cup of mixed greens (spinach, arugula, kale)

- 1/4 cup of diced cucumber

- 1/4 cup of cherry tomatoes, halved

- 1 tablespoon of extra virgin olive oil

- 1 tablespoon of lemon juice

- Salt and pepper to taste

- A sprinkle of dill for garnish

Instructions:

1. Grill or bake the salmon seasoned with salt and pepper until fully cooked and flaky. Set aside to cool.

2. In a large bowl, combine the cooked quinoa, mixed greens, cucumber, and cherry tomatoes.

3. Flake the cooled salmon and add it to the salad.

4. In a small bowl, whisk together the olive oil, lemon juice, salt, and pepper. Pour over the salad and toss to combine.

5. Garnish with dill before serving.

This meal is rich in omega-3 fatty acids, which are crucial for reducing inflammation and supporting hormonal balance. Quinoa provides a gluten-free source of fiber and protein, essential for gut health and satiety.

Anti-Inflammatory Turmeric Chicken and Vegetables

Ingredients:

- 2 chicken breasts, cut into bite-sized pieces
- 1 cup of broccoli florets
- 1 cup of sliced carrots
- 1/2 cup of red bell pepper, sliced
- 1 tablespoon of coconut oil
- 1 teaspoon of ground turmeric
- 1/2 teaspoon of ginger
- Salt and pepper to taste
- 1 tablespoon of apple cider vinegar
- 1 tablespoon of tamari or coconut aminos

Instructions:

1. Heat the coconut oil in a large skillet over medium heat. Add the chicken pieces, seasoning them with turmeric, ginger, salt, and pepper. Cook until the chicken is golden and cooked through.

2. Add the broccoli, carrots, and red bell pepper to the skillet. Stir-fry until the vegetables are tender but still crisp.

3. Drizzle the apple cider vinegar and tamari (or coconut aminos) over the chicken and vegetables, stirring well to combine.

4. Cook for an additional 2-3 minutes, allowing the flavors to meld.

This dish is packed with anti-inflammatory ingredients like turmeric and ginger, supporting thyroid health and reducing autoimmune reactions. The vegetables provide essential nutrients and fiber, while the chicken offers a lean protein source to stabilize blood sugar and support muscle repair.

Incorporating these recipes into your meal planning is a step towards building a resilient foundation for managing Hashimoto's. Consistency in consuming meals that support thyroid health and reduce inflammation can significantly decrease the likelihood of relapses, empowering you to maintain long-term well-being.

11.3 WORKBOOK EXERCISE: REFLECTION AND SETTING GOALS

Step 1: Create a dedicated section in your journal or digital document titled "Reflections and Future Goals."

Step 2: Reflect on the progress you've made over the past 12 weeks. List out the changes you've noticed in your symptoms, energy levels, and overall well-being. Be specific about any improvements or challenges you've encountered.

Step 3: Identify the strategies and habits that have been most beneficial to your healing journey. These could include dietary changes, stress reduction techniques, exercise routines, or supplements that have made a significant difference.

Step 4: Acknowledge any setbacks or areas where progress has been slower than expected. Consider what factors might have contributed to these challenges and how they can be addressed moving forward.

Step 5: Set specific, measurable goals for the next 3 months. These could relate to further dietary adjustments, incorporating new forms of exercise, deepening stress management practices, or exploring additional supportive therapies.

Step 6: Break down each goal into actionable steps. For example, if your goal is to improve gut health, your steps might include scheduling a consultation with a nutritionist, increasing your intake of fermented foods, and starting a food diary to track how different foods affect your symptoms.

Step 7: Schedule regular check-ins with yourself in your journal or digital document. These could be weekly or monthly, depending on what feels most supportive. Use these check-ins to assess your progress towards your goals, adjust your strategies as needed, and celebrate your successes.

Step 8: Consider any additional resources or support you might need to achieve your goals. This could include books, online courses, support groups, or professional guidance from healthcare providers specializing in Hashimoto's and thyroid health.

Step 9: Reflect on how your understanding of Hashimoto's and your body has evolved. Write down any new insights you've gained and how they will influence your approach to long-term maintenance.

Step 10: Reaffirm your commitment to your health and well-being. Write a short statement that reflects your dedication to continuing the practices that support your thyroid health and overall wellness.

Step 11: Keep your journal or digital document in a readily accessible place, ensuring that you can easily review and update your goals and reflections as you continue on your healing journey.

Part 4:
Advanced Tools and Resources

Chapter 12: Nutrition and Dietary Guidance

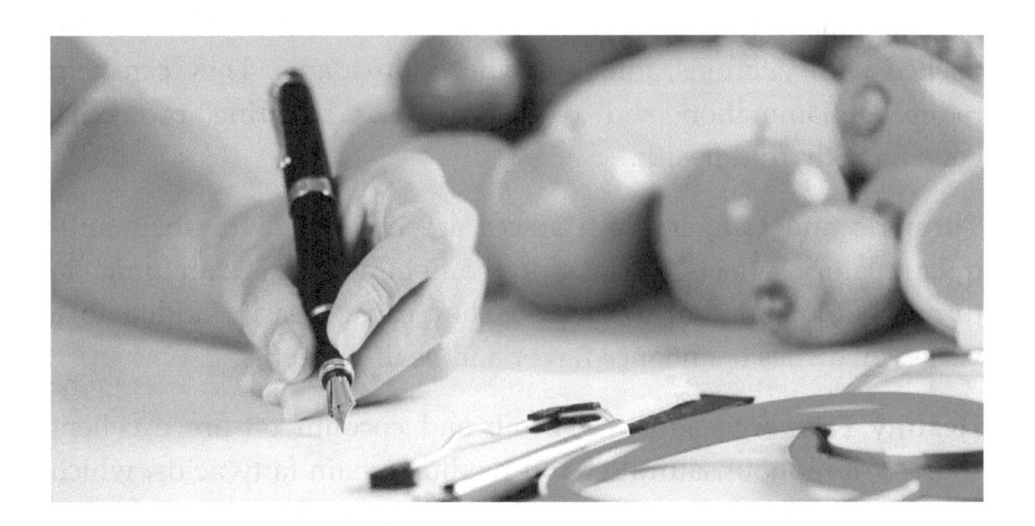

12.1: INTRODUCING ANTI-INFLAMMATORY FOODS

Inflammation plays a pivotal role in the progression of Hashimoto's thyroiditis, exacerbating symptoms and hindering the body's natural healing processes. By incorporating anti-inflammatory foods into your diet, you can significantly mitigate these effects, paving the way for improved thyroid health and overall well-being. The following is a detailed list of anti-inflammatory foods that should become staples in your nutritional regimen, accompanied by three recipes to seamlessly integrate these powerful ingredients into your daily meals.

Foods Rich in Omega-3 Fatty Acids: These are essential for combating inflammation. Sources include fatty fish like salmon, mackerel, and sardines, as well as flaxseeds, chia seeds, and walnuts. Incorporating these foods into your diet can help reduce the inflammatory markers associated with Hashimoto's.

Leafy Greens: Vegetables such as spinach, kale, and Swiss chard are high in antioxidants and polyphenols, known for their anti-inflammatory properties. These nutrients can help protect against cellular damage and support a healthy immune response.

Berries: Blueberries, strawberries, raspberries, and blackberries are packed with vitamins, minerals, and antioxidants. They can help reduce inflammation and oxidative stress, offering protective benefits to thyroid health.

Turmeric and Ginger: Both spices are renowned for their anti-inflammatory effects, thanks to compounds like curcumin in turmeric and gingerol in ginger. They can be easily added to a variety of dishes to enhance flavor and health benefits.

Healthy Fats: Avocados, olive oil, and coconut oil are excellent sources of monounsaturated and medium-chain fatty acids, which can help lower inflammation levels and improve hormone balance.

Recipe 1: Omega-3 Rich Salmon with Garlic Spinach

Ingredients:

- 4 salmon fillets
- 2 tablespoons olive oil
- 4 cups of fresh spinach
- 2 garlic cloves, minced
- Lemon wedges for serving
- Salt and pepper to taste

Instructions:

1. Preheat your oven to 400°F (200°C). Line a baking sheet with parchment paper.

2. Place salmon fillets on the prepared baking sheet. Drizzle with 1 tablespoon of olive oil, and season with salt and pepper. Bake for 12-15 minutes, or until salmon is cooked through.

3. While the salmon is baking, heat the remaining olive oil in a large skillet over medium heat. Add garlic and sauté for 1 minute. Add spinach and cook until wilted, about 3-4 minutes. Season with salt and pepper.

4. Serve the salmon with garlic spinach and a wedge of lemon.

Recipe 2: Anti-Inflammatory Berry Smoothie

Ingredients:

- 1 cup mixed berries (fresh or frozen)
- 1 banana
- 1 tablespoon chia seeds
- 1 cup spinach
- 1 cup almond milk or water
- A pinch of turmeric

Instructions:

1. Combine all ingredients in a blender.

2. Blend on high until smooth.

3. Serve immediately for a refreshing, anti-inflammatory boost.

Chapter 12:
Nutrition and Dietary Guidance

Recipe 3: Turmeric Ginger Tea

Ingredients:

- 1-inch piece of fresh turmeric, thinly sliced

- 1-inch piece of fresh ginger, thinly sliced

- 4 cups of water

- Honey to taste

Instructions:

1. Combine turmeric, ginger, and water in a saucepan. Bring to a boil.

2. Reduce heat and simmer for 10-15 minutes.

3. Strain the tea into cups. Add honey to taste and enjoy warm.

By integrating these anti-inflammatory foods and recipes into your diet, you can support your body's natural defenses against Hashimoto's thyroiditis, reduce inflammation, and promote a state of balance and healing. Remember, consistency is key to seeing and maintaining results, so aim to include these foods and meals regularly as part of your overall health strategy.

12.2: COOKING WITHOUT INFLAMMATORY OILS

Choosing healthier oils for cooking is a crucial step in reducing inflammation and supporting your thyroid health. Many common cooking oils, such as vegetable oil and canola oil, are high in omega-6 fatty acids, which can contribute to inflammation when consumed in excess. Opting for oils with a better balance of omega-3 to omega-6 fatty acids, or those with anti-inflammatory properties, can make a significant difference in your overall well-being.

Coconut Oil: This oil is rich in medium-chain triglycerides (MCTs), which are metabolized differently than other fats. They are known to boost metabolism and provide a quick source of energy. Coconut oil can withstand high cooking temperatures, making it ideal for sautéing and baking.

Extra Virgin Olive Oil: Packed with monounsaturated fats and antioxidants, extra virgin olive oil is a staple in anti-inflammatory diets. It's best used for low to medium heat cooking or added to dishes after cooking to preserve its health benefits.

Avocado Oil: With a high smoke point, avocado oil is versatile for cooking while being rich in monounsaturated fats and vitamin E, both known for their anti-inflammatory properties. It's suitable for frying, roasting, and even baking.

Grass-Fed Butter or Ghee: For those not sensitive to dairy, grass-fed butter and ghee (clarified butter) can be good options. They contain butyrate, a short-chain fatty acid that can help reduce inflammation and improve gut health.

Flaxseed Oil: Although not suitable for cooking due to its low smoke point, flaxseed oil is excellent for adding to salads or dishes after cooking. It's rich in ALA, a type of omega-3 fatty acid that fights inflammation.

Walnut Oil: Like flaxseed oil, walnut oil has a low smoke point and is best used in dressings or added to dishes after cooking. It's high in omega-3 fatty acids and antioxidants.

Sesame Oil: While it should be used sparingly due to its relatively high omega-6 content, sesame oil can add a burst of flavor to dishes. It's best to use it in low-heat cooking or add it to dishes after they've been cooked.

Recipe 1: Avocado Oil Roasted Brussels Sprouts

Ingredients:

- 1 lb Brussels sprouts, trimmed and halved
- 2 tablespoons avocado oil
- Salt and pepper to taste
- 2 cloves garlic, minced
- 1 teaspoon balsamic vinegar

Instructions:

1. Preheat your oven to 400°F (200°C).

2. Toss the Brussels sprouts with avocado oil, salt, and pepper on a baking sheet.

3. Roast for 20-25 minutes until tender and caramelized, stirring halfway through.

4. In the last 5 minutes of roasting, add the minced garlic to the pan.

5. Remove from oven and drizzle with balsamic vinegar before serving.

Recipe 2: Coconut Oil Stir-Fry with Vegetables and Chicken

Ingredients:

- 1 tablespoon coconut oil

- 1 lb chicken breast, thinly sliced

- 2 cups of mixed vegetables (bell peppers, broccoli, carrots)

- 2 cloves garlic, minced

- 1 tablespoon ginger, minced

- 2 tablespoons tamari or coconut aminos

- 1 teaspoon sesame seeds (optional)

Instructions:

1. Heat coconut oil in a large skillet or wok over medium-high heat.

2. Add chicken slices, cooking until golden and cooked through. Remove chicken and set aside.

3. In the same skillet, add another teaspoon of coconut oil if needed. Stir-fry the vegetables, garlic, and ginger until just tender.

4. Return the chicken to the skillet. Add tamari or coconut aminos, stirring to combine and heat through.

5. Garnish with sesame seeds before serving.

Incorporating these oils into your diet and using them in your cooking can help reduce inflammation and support your journey to healing Hashimoto's. Remember, the quality of the oil matters, so always opt for cold-pressed, unrefined oils when possible to maximize health benefits.

12.3: ANTI-INFLAMMATORY SPICES

Incorporating anti-inflammatory spices into your daily meals can significantly reduce inflammation and support thyroid health. Spices such as **turmeric, ginger, cinnamon,** and **black pepper** not only enhance the flavor of your dishes but also offer potent anti-inflammatory benefits. These spices contain compounds that have been shown to inhibit the production of inflammatory cytokines, providing natural relief from the autoimmune responses associated with Hashimoto's.

Turmeric, known for its active compound curcumin, has been widely studied for its anti-inflammatory, antioxidant, and anti-carcinogenic properties. To increase its bioavailability, it's recommended to combine turmeric with **black pepper**, which contains piperine, a natural substance that enhances the absorption of curcumin by 2000%.

Ginger, another powerful spice, contains gingerol, a substance with potent anti-inflammatory and antioxidant effects. Ginger can help reduce nausea and pain, including menstrual pain, which is particularly beneficial for those with Hashimoto's experiencing these symptoms.

Cinnamon is not only delicious but also packed with antioxidants that have anti-inflammatory effects. It can help lower blood sugar levels and reduce heart disease risk factors, making it a great addition to meals for those managing Hashimoto's.

To incorporate these spices into your diet, here are two recipes that are not only easy to prepare but also packed with anti-inflammatory benefits:

Golden Turmeric Latte

Ingredients:

- 1 cup almond milk
- 1 teaspoon turmeric powder
- 1/4 teaspoon ginger powder
- 1/4 teaspoon cinnamon powder
- A pinch of black pepper
- 1 teaspoon honey or maple syrup (optional)

Instructions:

1. Heat the almond milk in a small pot over medium heat until it's warm but not boiling.

2. Add the turmeric, ginger, cinnamon, and black pepper to the milk, whisking to combine.

3. Allow the mixture to simmer gently for a few minutes to infuse the flavors.

4. Remove from heat and sweeten with honey or maple syrup if desired.

5. Pour into a mug and enjoy warm.

Anti-Inflammatory Smoothie Bowl

Ingredients:

- 1 banana, frozen
- 1/2 cup mixed berries, frozen
- 1 tablespoon flaxseeds
- 1/2 teaspoon turmeric powder
- 1/4 teaspoon ginger powder
- A pinch of black pepper
- 1/2 cup spinach
- 1 cup almond milk or water
- Toppings: sliced banana, berries, chia seeds, and a sprinkle of cinnamon

Instructions:

1. In a blender, combine the banana, mixed berries, flaxseeds, turmeric, ginger, black pepper, spinach, and almond milk or water.

2. Blend on high until smooth and creamy.

3. Pour the smoothie into a bowl and add your desired toppings.

4. Enjoy immediately for a nutrient-packed meal that fights inflammation.

By integrating these spices and recipes into your daily routine, you can enjoy delicious meals while naturally reducing inflammation and supporting your journey to healing Hashimoto's. Remember, small dietary changes can make a significant impact on your overall health, and incorporating anti-inflammatory spices is an easy and effective step towards managing your symptoms.

Chapter 13: Nutritional Building Blocks for Thyroid Health

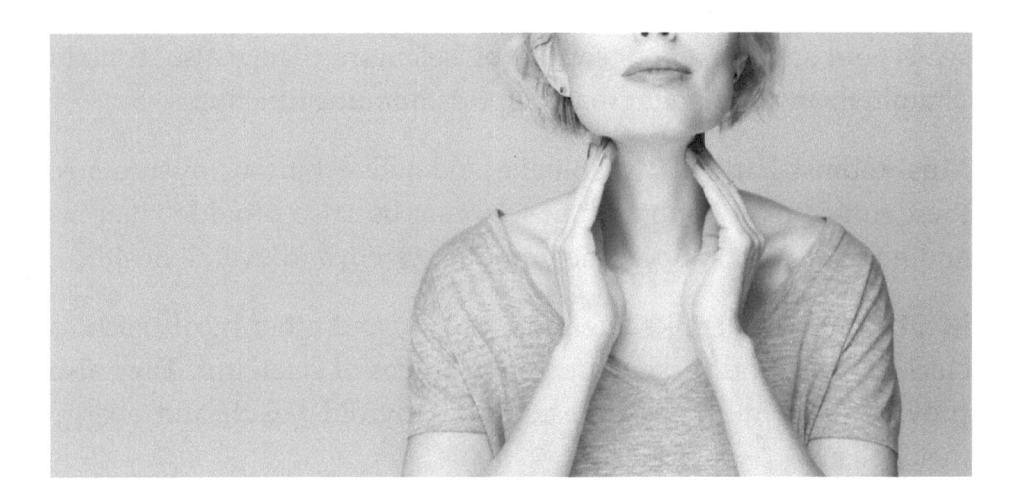

13.1: Selenium-Rich Foods

Selenium plays a crucial role in thyroid function by aiding in the production of thyroid hormones and protecting the thyroid gland from damage caused by oxidative stress. This trace mineral is essential for individuals with Hashimoto's to support overall thyroid health and immune function. Foods rich in selenium are an integral part of a diet aimed at managing Hashimoto's symptoms and promoting healing. Including selenium-rich foods in your daily intake can help balance thyroid function and reduce inflammation.

Brazil Nuts: One of the most potent sources of selenium, just one or two Brazil nuts can provide the daily recommended intake of selenium. They are easy to incorporate into your diet as a snack or chopped and sprinkled over salads.

Seafood: Fish such as tuna, halibut, and sardines, along with shellfish like shrimp and crab, are excellent sources of selenium. These not only provide the necessary mineral but also omega-3 fatty acids, beneficial for reducing inflammation.

Eggs: Eggs are a versatile food that can contribute significantly to your daily selenium intake. They also offer high-quality protein and other essential nutrients beneficial for thyroid health.

Sunflower Seeds: A great snack option or salad topping, sunflower seeds are another good source of selenium. They also contain vitamin E, an antioxidant that supports immune function.

Mushrooms: Particularly shiitake and white button mushrooms, these fungi are not only rich in selenium but also provide vitamins and minerals that support the immune system and overall health.

Meat: Organ meats like liver and kidney, and other meats such as chicken, beef, and turkey, are good sources of selenium. They also provide other nutrients necessary for thyroid health and energy metabolism.

To incorporate selenium into your diet effectively, consider the following recipes that utilize these selenium-rich ingredients:

Recipe 1: Selenium-Boosting Snack Mix

Ingredients:

- 1 cup Brazil nuts
- 1/2 cup sunflower seeds
- 1/2 cup dried shiitake mushrooms, chopped
- 1 tablespoon olive oil
- Sea salt to taste
- 1 teaspoon garlic powder

Instructions:

1. Preheat the oven to 300°F (150°C).

2. In a bowl, mix Brazil nuts, sunflower seeds, and dried shiitake mushrooms with olive oil, sea salt, and garlic powder until evenly coated.

3. Spread the mix on a baking sheet in a single layer.

4. Bake for 10-15 minutes or until lightly toasted, stirring halfway through.

5. Let it cool before serving. Store in an airtight container.

Recipe 2: Simple Tuna and Avocado Salad

Ingredients:

- 1 can (4 ounces) tuna in water, drained
- 1 ripe avocado, diced
- 1/2 cup chopped cucumber
- 1/4 cup diced red onion
- 2 tablespoons chopped cilantro
- Juice of 1 lime
- Salt and pepper to taste
- Mixed greens for serving

Instructions:

1. In a bowl, combine the tuna, avocado, cucumber, red onion, and cilantro.

2. Add lime juice, salt, and pepper. Gently toss to combine.

3. Serve over a bed of mixed greens for a refreshing and nutritious meal.

Incorporating selenium-rich foods into your diet is a straightforward and effective way to support your thyroid health and overall well-being. These recipes are designed to be simple, delicious, and packed with nutrients critical for managing Hashimoto's. Regular consumption of these foods, in combination with other lifestyle and dietary adjustments outlined in this workbook, can significantly contribute to your healing journey.

13.2: Zinc-Rich Foods and Recipes

Zinc plays a pivotal role in thyroid function and overall immune health, making it an essential nutrient for individuals dealing with Hashimoto's thyroiditis. This mineral helps in the enzymatic reactions necessary for thyroid hormone synthesis and metabolism, and it supports the immune system's balance, reducing the likelihood of autoimmune flare-ups. Foods rich in zinc include a variety of sources, ensuring that individuals with different dietary preferences can incorporate this nutrient into their meals effectively.

Oysters: Known as one of the highest sources of zinc, oysters can significantly boost your intake with just a few servings per week. They also provide a good amount of protein and omega-3 fatty acids.

Beef: Grass-fed beef is not only a rich source of high-quality protein but also contains high levels of zinc, making it a beneficial addition to the diet for supporting thyroid health.

Pumpkin Seeds: For a plant-based zinc option, pumpkin seeds are an excellent choice. They can be easily added to salads, yogurts, or simply enjoyed as a snack.

Lentils: Another plant-based source, lentils, are not only rich in zinc but also provide fiber, protein, and other minerals essential for maintaining a healthy thyroid function.

Spinach: This leafy green is a versatile vegetable that can be easily incorporated into your diet and is a good plant-based source of zinc.

Recipe 1: Zinc-Boosting Beef Stir-Fry

Ingredients:

- 1 lb grass-fed beef, thinly sliced
- 2 tablespoons coconut oil
- 1 bell pepper, sliced
- 1 zucchini, sliced
- 2 cloves garlic, minced
- 1 tablespoon ginger, minced
- 1/4 cup tamari or soy sauce
- 1 tablespoon sesame oil
- 2 tablespoons pumpkin seeds for garnish

Instructions:

1. Heat one tablespoon of coconut oil in a large skillet over medium-high heat. Add the beef slices and cook until browned. Remove from the skillet and set aside.

2. In the same skillet, add the remaining coconut oil, bell pepper, zucchini, garlic, and ginger. Stir-fry for about 5 minutes, or until the vegetables are tender but still crisp.

3. Return the beef to the skillet and add tamari or soy sauce. Cook for an additional 2-3 minutes, stirring to combine all the ingredients well.

4. Drizzle with sesame oil and garnish with pumpkin seeds before serving.

Recipe 2: Lentil and Spinach Salad

Ingredients:

- 1 cup lentils, cooked and cooled

- 2 cups spinach, roughly chopped

- 1/2 cucumber, diced

- 1/4 cup red onion, finely chopped

- 2 tablespoons olive oil

- Juice of 1 lemon

- Salt and pepper to taste

- 1/4 cup feta cheese, crumbled (optional)

Instructions:

1. In a large bowl, combine the cooked lentils, spinach, cucumber, and red onion.

2. In a small bowl, whisk together the olive oil, lemon juice, salt, and pepper. Pour the dressing over the salad and toss to combine.

3. Sprinkle with feta cheese if using, and serve chilled or at room temperature.

Incorporating zinc into your diet through these foods and recipes can help support your thyroid health and overall well-being as part of your journey with Hashimoto's. Regular consumption of these zinc-rich options, along with other nutrient-dense foods, can contribute to a balanced and healthy diet that supports the management of Hashimoto's symptoms.

13.3: Vitamin D and Iodine Sources

Vitamin D and iodine are essential nutrients for thyroid health, playing pivotal roles in hormone production and regulation. Deficiencies in either can exacerbate symptoms of Hashimoto's thyroiditis and impair overall well-being. Fortunately, incorporating sources of these nutrients into your diet can be both simple and delicious.

Vitamin D is famously known as the "sunshine vitamin" because the body can produce it when exposed to sunlight. However, food sources also contribute to meeting your daily requirement. Fatty fish like salmon, mackerel, and sardines are excellent sources, as are egg yolks and fortified foods such as milk, orange juice, and cereals.

Iodine is crucial for thyroid function as it is a key component of thyroid hormones. Seafood is a rich source of iodine, particularly seaweed, cod, and shrimp. Dairy products, eggs, and iodized salt are also good sources. It's important to consume iodine in moderation, as both too little and too much can lead to thyroid problems.

Recipe 1: Salmon with Roasted Vegetables

Ingredients:

- 4 salmon fillets
- 2 tablespoons olive oil
- 1 teaspoon garlic powder
- Salt and pepper to taste
- 1 cup cherry tomatoes
- 1 zucchini, sliced
- 1 yellow squash, sliced
- 1 tablespoon fresh dill, chopped

Instructions:

1. Preheat your oven to 400°F (200°C).

2. Place the salmon fillets on a baking sheet lined with parchment paper.

3. Drizzle olive oil over the salmon and vegetables. Sprinkle garlic powder, salt, and pepper, ensuring all pieces are well-seasoned.

4. Scatter the cherry tomatoes, zucchini, and yellow squash around the salmon.

5. Roast in the oven for 20-25 minutes or until the salmon is cooked through and the vegetables are tender.

6. Garnish with fresh dill before serving.

This recipe provides a hearty dose of vitamin D through the salmon and a variety of nutrients from the colorful vegetables.

Recipe 2: Seaweed Salad with Sesame Dressing

Ingredients:

- 2 cups dried seaweed (wakame)
- 3 tablespoons soy sauce
- 2 tablespoons sesame oil
- 1 tablespoon rice vinegar
- 1 teaspoon honey
- 1/2 teaspoon grated ginger
- 1 tablespoon sesame seeds
- 1/2 cucumber, thinly sliced
- 1 carrot, julienned

Instructions:

1. Rehydrate the dried seaweed in water for about 15 minutes, then drain well.

2. In a bowl, whisk together soy sauce, sesame oil, rice vinegar, honey, and grated ginger to create the dressing.

3. Toss the rehydrated seaweed with the cucumber and carrot in the dressing until evenly coated.

4. Sprinkle sesame seeds over the salad before serving.

Seaweed is an outstanding source of iodine, and this salad is a refreshing way to include it in your diet.

Chapter 14: Gut Health and Hormonal Balance

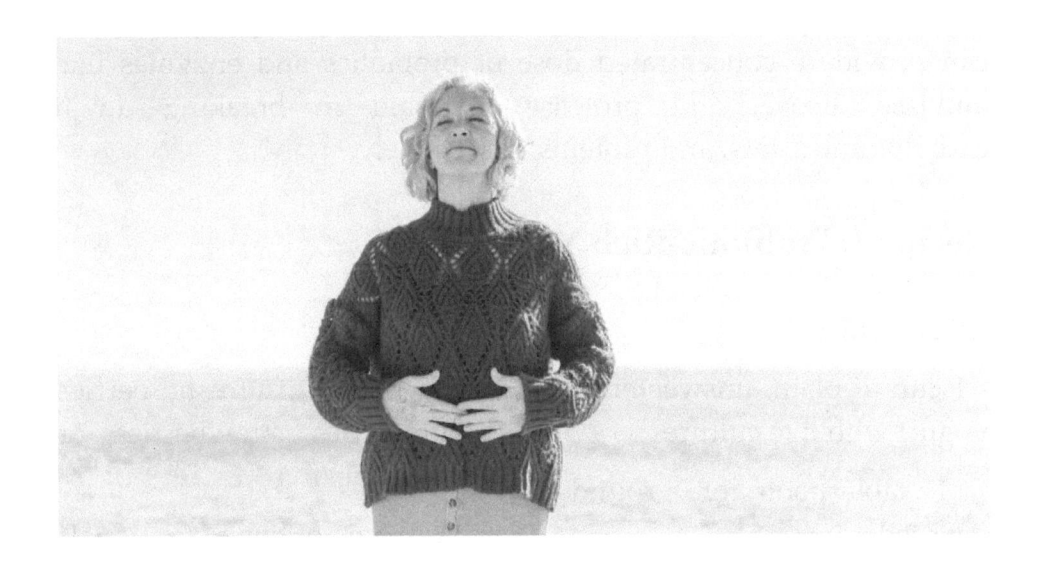

14.1: PROBIOTIC FOODS AND DIGESTIVE ENZYMES

Incorporating probiotic-rich foods into your diet is a cornerstone of supporting gut health, particularly for individuals managing Hashimoto's thyroiditis. Probiotics, the beneficial bacteria found in certain foods, play a crucial role in maintaining a healthy gut microbiome, which in turn can influence overall health and hormonal balance. Alongside probiotics, digestive enzymes are essential for optimizing nutrient absorption and digestion, further supporting gut integrity and function.

Chapter 14:
Gut Health and Hormonal Balance

Fermented Foods: A primary source of natural probiotics. Examples include yogurt with live cultures, kefir, sauerkraut, kimchi, miso, and kombucha. These foods introduce beneficial bacteria to the digestive tract, aiding in digestion and the absorption of nutrients.

Prebiotic Foods: While not containing probiotics themselves, prebiotic foods support the growth of beneficial gut bacteria. Foods such as garlic, onions, leeks, asparagus, bananas, and chicory root feed healthy gut flora, promoting a balanced gut microbiome.

Supplementation: In some cases, dietary sources of probiotics and digestive enzymes may not be sufficient. High-quality supplements can provide a concentrated dose of probiotics and enzymes like amylase, lipase, and protease that aid in breaking down carbohydrates, fats, and proteins, respectively.

Recipe 1: Probiotic-Rich Yogurt Bowl

Ingredients:

- 1 cup of plain, unsweetened yogurt with live cultures
- 1 tablespoon of ground flaxseed
- ½ cup of fresh berries (blueberries, strawberries, or raspberries)
- A drizzle of honey (optional)

Instructions:

1. In a bowl, combine the yogurt and ground flaxseed.

2. Top with fresh berries and a drizzle of honey if desired.

3. Enjoy as a nourishing breakfast or snack that supports gut health.

Recipe 2: Homemade Sauerkraut

Ingredients:

- 1 medium cabbage, finely shredded
- 1.5 tablespoons of sea salt
- Clean, filtered water

Instructions:

1. In a large bowl, mix the shredded cabbage with sea salt, massaging the salt into the cabbage until it starts to release water.

2. Pack the cabbage tightly into a clean jar, pressing down until the water rises above the cabbage. Leave about 2 inches of space at the top.

3. Seal the jar with a tight lid. Let it sit at room temperature for at least 2 weeks, checking periodically to ensure the cabbage remains submerged in water.

4. Once fermented, store in the refrigerator to slow down the fermentation process.

Recipe 3: Kefir Smoothie

Ingredients:

- 1 cup of kefir
- ½ banana
- ½ cup of mixed frozen berries
- A handful of spinach
- 1 tablespoon of chia seeds

Instructions:

1. Combine all ingredients in a blender.

2. Blend until smooth.

3. Enjoy immediately for a probiotic-rich, nutrient-packed drink.

By integrating these probiotic and enzyme-rich foods into your diet, you can support your gut health, which is instrumental in managing

Hashimoto's thyroiditis. Remember, a healthy gut contributes to a healthy body and can significantly impact your healing journey.

14.2: Foods for Cortisol Management and Balanced Meals

Managing cortisol levels is essential for those dealing with Hashimoto's, as elevated cortisol can exacerbate symptoms and hinder the healing process. Consuming a diet focused on balancing hormones can significantly impact your well-being. Foods rich in antioxidants, omega-3 fatty acids, and phytonutrients play a pivotal role in moderating stress responses and supporting adrenal health. Including a variety of whole foods like leafy greens, fatty fish, nuts, and seeds can provide the necessary nutrients to help regulate cortisol levels and promote hormonal balance.

Foods That Help Manage Cortisol:

- **Leafy Greens**: Spinach, kale, and Swiss chard are loaded with magnesium, a mineral that aids in cortisol regulation.

- **Fatty Fish**: Salmon, mackerel, and sardines are high in omega-3 fatty acids, which have been shown to reduce stress markers.

- **Nuts and Seeds**: Almonds, flaxseeds, and chia seeds are not only great sources of healthy fats but also contain magnesium.

- **Berries**: Blueberries, strawberries, and raspberries are rich in antioxidants that help reduce stress-related inflammation.

- **Avocados**: High in fiber, potassium, and healthy fats, avocados can help lower blood pressure and cortisol levels.

Recipe 1: Omega-3 Rich Salmon Salad

Ingredients:

- 4 ounces of wild-caught salmon
- 2 cups of mixed greens (spinach, arugula, kale)
- 1/4 avocado, sliced
- 1/2 cup of cooked quinoa
- A handful of walnuts
- Dressing: 2 tablespoons of extra virgin olive oil, 1 tablespoon of lemon juice, salt, and pepper to taste

Instructions:

1. Grill or bake the salmon to your preference.

2. In a large bowl, toss the mixed greens, avocado slices, and cooked quinoa.

3. Top the salad with the cooked salmon and a handful of walnuts.

4. Whisk together the olive oil, lemon juice, salt, and pepper for the dressing.

5. Drizzle the dressing over the salad and serve.

This meal combines the stress-reducing benefits of omega-3 fatty acids, magnesium, and antioxidants, making it a perfect choice for managing cortisol levels.

Recipe 2: Stress-Reducing Berry Smoothie

Ingredients:

- 1 cup of mixed berries (blueberries, strawberries, raspberries)
- 1 banana
- 1 tablespoon of chia seeds
- 1 cup of spinach
- 1 cup of almond milk or water
- A handful of almonds

Chapter 14: Gut Health and Hormonal Balance

Instructions:

1. Combine the mixed berries, banana, chia seeds, spinach, and almond milk or water in a blender.

2. Blend until smooth.

3. Pour into a glass and garnish with a handful of almonds for an extra magnesium boost.

This smoothie is not only delicious but also packed with nutrients that aid in cortisol management and overall hormonal balance. The inclusion of spinach and chia seeds adds a magnesium boost, while the berries provide antioxidants to combat stress-related inflammation.

Incorporating these foods and recipes into your diet can help manage cortisol levels, supporting your journey to heal Hashimoto's. Remember, a balanced approach to nutrition, focusing on whole, nutrient-dense foods, is key to restoring energy, losing weight, and achieving hormonal harmony.

Chapter 15: Recipes and Meal Planning Tools

15.1: Easy Breakfast Recipes

Recipe 1: Simple Avocado Toast

Ingredients:

- 1 ripe avocado
- 2 slices of whole grain bread
- Salt to taste
- Pepper to taste
- Red pepper flakes (optional)
- 1 teaspoon of lemon juice
- Fresh herbs (optional, such as cilantro or parsley)

Instructions:

Step 1: Toast the two slices of whole grain bread to your preference using a toaster or a skillet over medium heat.

Step 2: While the bread is toasting, cut the avocado in half and remove the pit. Scoop out the avocado flesh into a bowl.

Step 3: Add the teaspoon of lemon juice to the avocado. This not only adds flavor but also helps in keeping the avocado from browning quickly.

Step 4: Using a fork, mash the avocado until it's smooth with some small chunks remaining for texture.

Step 5: Season the mashed avocado with salt and pepper to taste. If you enjoy a bit of spice, add a sprinkle of red pepper flakes as well.

Step 6: Once the bread is toasted to your liking, spread the mashed avocado evenly over each slice.

Step 7: If desired, add a garnish of fresh herbs on top for an extra burst of flavor and a touch of elegance.

Step 8: Serve immediately and enjoy as a nutritious and energizing start to your day.

Nutritional Note: Avocado is a great source of healthy fats, fiber, and various essential nutrients, making it an excellent choice for those looking to support thyroid health and overall well-being. Whole grain bread adds a beneficial dose of fiber and energy-sustaining complex carbohydrates.

Recipe 2: Quick Oatmeal with Berries

Ingredients Needed:

- 1/2 cup of rolled oats
- 1 cup of water or milk (almond, soy, or dairy, based on your preference)
- Pinch of salt
- 1/2 cup of mixed berries (fresh or frozen)
- 1 tablespoon of chia seeds
- 1 tablespoon of honey or maple syrup (optional)
- 1/4 teaspoon of cinnamon (optional)

Instructions:

1. **Preparation:** Gather all the ingredients. If using frozen berries, consider setting them out to thaw slightly as you prepare the oatmeal.

2. **Cooking the Oats:** In a small saucepan, bring the 1 cup of water or milk to a boil. Add a pinch of salt.

3. **Adding Oats:** Stir in the 1/2 cup of rolled oats. Reduce the heat to medium-low and cook for 5 minutes, stirring occasionally to prevent sticking. If you prefer a thinner consistency, you can add a little more water or milk.

4. **Mixing in Flavors:** While the oatmeal is still on the stove, add the cinnamon if you're using it. This is also a good time to stir in the honey or maple syrup for sweetness.

5. **Incorporating Berries:** Once the oatmeal is cooked to your liking, remove it from the heat. Gently fold in the mixed berries and chia seeds. The heat from the oatmeal will slightly soften the berries and allow the chia seeds to begin to gel, adding a nice texture.

6. **Serving:** Transfer the cooked oatmeal into a bowl. If desired, sprinkle a little more cinnamon on top, or add a few more berries for decoration.

7. **Adjustments:** Taste the oatmeal and adjust the sweetness if necessary. Depending on your dietary preferences, you can also top it with a dollop of Greek yogurt for extra protein or a sprinkle of nuts for healthy fats.

8. **Enjoy:** Enjoy your quick oatmeal with berries as a nourishing start to your day, knowing it's not just delicious but also supportive of your thyroid health.

Note: This recipe is customizable based on dietary needs and preferences. Feel free to substitute ingredients as needed to align with your health goals and dietary restrictions.

Chapter 15:
Recipes and Meal Planning Tools

Recipe 3: Easy Greek Yogurt Parfait

Ingredients:

- 1 cup plain Greek yogurt

- 2 tablespoons honey or pure maple syrup

- ½ cup granola (look for a low-sugar, high-fiber option)

- ½ cup mixed berries (such as strawberries, blueberries, and raspberries)

- 1 tablespoon chia seeds (optional)

- 1 tablespoon sliced almonds (optional)

Instructions:

Step 1: Choose a tall glass or a mason jar for layering your parfait. This not only makes the parfait visually appealing but also makes it easy to transport if you're on the go.

Step 2: Begin by placing a layer of Greek yogurt at the bottom of your chosen container. Aim for about a third of the yogurt you've prepared.

Step 3: Drizzle a portion of the honey or maple syrup over the yogurt. Adjust the sweetness according to your preference, but remember, natural sweetness from the berries will also add to the overall flavor.

Step 4: Add a layer of granola over the yogurt and sweetener. This will add a satisfying crunch to your parfait. If you're adding chia seeds, sprinkle a teaspoon over the granola.

Step 5: Add a layer of mixed berries. The more colorful, the better. These berries are not only delicious but are packed with antioxidants and vitamins that are beneficial for your health.

Step 6: Repeat the layering process until all ingredients are used up, finishing with a layer of berries on top. For an extra touch of flavor and texture, sprinkle sliced almonds and a final drizzle of honey or maple syrup over the final layer.

Step 7: If you've included chia seeds in your layers, allow the parfait to sit for a few minutes before eating. Chia seeds absorb liquid and will help thicken the yogurt, making the parfait creamier.

Step 8: Enjoy immediately, or cover and refrigerate if you're preparing this as a make-ahead breakfast. The parfait can be stored in the refrigerator for up to a day, though keep in mind the granola may soften over time.

Nutritional Tip: Greek yogurt is a fantastic source of protein, which is essential for tissue repair and muscle maintenance. Choosing plain Greek yogurt over flavored varieties helps reduce added sugar intake, aligning with a diet that supports thyroid health and overall well-being.

Recipe 4: Basic Smoothie Bowl

Ingredients:

- 1/2 cup unsweetened almond milk (or any plant-based milk of your choice)

- 1/4 cup frozen blueberries

- 1/4 cup frozen strawberries

- 1/2 banana, sliced and frozen

- 1 tablespoon chia seeds

- 1 tablespoon flaxseed meal

- 1 scoop of your preferred protein powder (ensure it's gluten-free and fits Hashimoto's dietary recommendations)

- A handful of spinach leaves (for an iron and fiber boost)

- Optional toppings: sliced almonds, coconut flakes, fresh fruit slices, or a drizzle of honey

Chapter 15: Recipes and Meal Planning Tools

Instructions:

1. **Prepare Ingredients:** Ensure all your fruits are properly washed, sliced, and frozen. Pre-freezing the fruits ensures a thick and creamy texture for your smoothie bowl.

2. **Blend:** In a high-speed blender, combine the almond milk, frozen blueberries, frozen strawberries, frozen banana slices, chia seeds, flaxseed meal, protein powder, and spinach leaves. Blend on high until the mixture is smooth and creamy. If the mixture is too thick, you can add a little more almond milk to reach your desired consistency.

3. **Taste Test:** Before proceeding to the next step, taste your smoothie mix. If you prefer a bit of sweetness, you can add a drizzle of honey or maple syrup and blend again for a few seconds.

4. **Serve:** Pour the smoothie mixture into a bowl. Use a spatula to smooth the top. The consistency should be thick enough to hold your toppings in place.

5. **Add Toppings:** Sprinkle your chosen toppings over the smoothie bowl. This can include sliced almonds for crunch, coconut flakes for a hint of sweetness, fresh fruit slices for added vitamins, or a drizzle of honey for natural sweetness.

6. **Enjoy Immediately:** Smoothie bowls are best enjoyed fresh. Use a spoon to enjoy the creamy texture along with the crunchy and fresh toppings.

Tip: Experiment with different fruit combinations and toppings to keep your breakfast exciting and nutritious. Remember, managing Hashimoto's is about finding what works best for your body while ensuring you're nourishing it with the right nutrients.

Recipe 5: Classic Scrambled Eggs

Ingredients:

- 2 large eggs

- 1 tablespoon of olive oil or coconut oil

- Salt and pepper to taste

- Optional: 1/4 cup of chopped vegetables (spinach, bell peppers, onions)

- Optional: 1 tablespoon of shredded cheese (choose a dairy-free option if necessary)

Instructions:

Step 1: Crack the eggs into a bowl. Add salt and pepper to taste. If you're including vegetables or cheese, add them into the bowl as well.

Step 2: Beat the eggs and optional ingredients together until the mixture is uniform in color and texture.

Step 3: Heat a non-stick skillet over medium heat. Add the olive oil or coconut oil to the skillet, ensuring the surface is fully coated to prevent sticking.

Step 4: Once the oil is hot, pour the egg mixture into the skillet. Let it sit without stirring for about 20 seconds or until the edges start to set.

Step 5: With a spatula, gently stir the eggs from the outside toward the center, forming large soft curds.

Step 6: Continue cooking, stirring occasionally, until the eggs are fully cooked but still moist and no visible liquid egg remains.

Step 7: Remove the skillet from heat. If you've opted for cheese, sprinkle it over the eggs now so it can melt into the warm mixture.

Step 8: Serve immediately on a plate. For a balanced meal, consider pairing the scrambled eggs with a side of whole-grain toast and fresh fruit.

Nutritional Note: Eggs are a great source of high-quality protein and contain essential nutrients beneficial for thyroid health, such as iodine and selenium. Opting for added vegetables can increase the fiber content, which supports healthy digestion and nutrient absorption.

15.2: Easy Lunch Recipes

Recipe 6: Grilled Chicken Salad

Ingredients:

- 1 boneless, skinless chicken breast (about 6 oz)
- Salt and pepper to taste
- 1 tablespoon olive oil
- 2 cups mixed greens (such as arugula, spinach, and romaine)
- 1/2 cup cherry tomatoes, halved
- 1/4 cucumber, sliced
- 1/4 red onion, thinly sliced
- 1/4 avocado, sliced
- 2 tablespoons balsamic vinaigrette (look for a low-sugar option or make your own)

Instructions:

Step 1: Season the chicken breast with salt and pepper on both sides.

Step 2: Heat olive oil in a grill pan or skillet over medium-high heat. Once hot, add the chicken breast.

Step 3: Cook the chicken for 6-7 minutes on each side, or until fully cooked through and no longer pink in the center. The internal temperature should reach 165°F.

Step 4: Remove the chicken from the pan and let it rest for a few minutes. Then, slice it into strips.

Step 5: In a large bowl, combine the mixed greens, cherry tomatoes, cucumber, and red onion.

Step 6: Add the sliced chicken on top of the salad.

Step 7: Add the avocado slices to the salad.

Step 8: Drizzle the balsamic vinaigrette over the salad.

Step 9: Gently toss the salad to mix the ingredients and evenly coat with the dressing.

Step 10: Serve immediately.

Nutritional Note: This salad combines lean protein from the chicken with a variety of vegetables, offering a rich source of vitamins, minerals, and antioxidants. The olive oil and avocado provide healthy fats, beneficial for hormone balance and inflammation reduction.

Chapter 15:
Recipes and Meal Planning Tools

Recipe 7: Veggie Wrap with Hummus

Ingredients:

- 1 large whole grain tortilla wrap
- 2 tablespoons of hummus
- 1/4 cup of grated carrots
- 1/4 cup of sliced cucumber
- 1/4 cup of red bell pepper strips
- 1/4 cup of spinach leaves
- 1/4 avocado, sliced
- Salt and pepper to taste
- Optional: a sprinkle of chili flakes for extra spice

Instructions:

Step 1: Lay the whole grain tortilla wrap flat on a clean surface. Ensure it's at room temperature to prevent tearing when you add the fillings and roll it up.

Step 2: Spread the hummus evenly over the tortilla, leaving about an inch from the edge to help with rolling and to prevent the hummus from squeezing out.

Step 3: On one side of the tortilla, arrange the grated carrots, sliced cucumber, red bell pepper strips, and spinach leaves in neat, compact rows. This not only makes the wrap visually appealing but also ensures you get a bit of each flavor in every bite.

Step 4: Add the avocado slices on top of the arranged vegetables. The avocado adds a creamy texture that complements the crunch of the veggies.

Step 5: Season with salt and pepper to taste. If you like a bit of spice, sprinkle some chili flakes over the vegetables.

Step 6: Carefully start rolling the tortilla from the side with the fillings, tucking in the edges as you go to keep the fillings secure. Roll as tightly as possible without tearing the tortilla.

Step 7: Once rolled, use a sharp knife to cut the wrap in half diagonally. This makes it easier to eat and also displays the colorful cross-section of the veggies and hummus.

Step 8: Serve immediately, or wrap tightly in parchment paper or aluminum foil for a convenient, portable lunch option.

Nutritional Note: This veggie wrap with hummus is not only delicious but packed with nutrients essential for thyroid health, including fiber from the vegetables and healthy fats from the avocado and hummus. Whole grain tortillas are a great source of complex carbohydrates, providing sustained energy throughout the day.

Recipe 8: Quinoa and Black Bean Bowl

Ingredients:

- 1 cup quinoa
- 2 cups water or vegetable broth
- 1 can (15 ounces) black beans, drained and rinsed
- 1 medium red bell pepper, diced
- 1 medium avocado, diced
- 1/2 cup fresh cilantro, chopped
- 1/4 cup red onion, finely chopped
- 1 lime, juiced
- 2 tablespoons olive oil
- Salt and pepper to taste
- Optional: 1 teaspoon ground cumin
- Optional: 1/2 teaspoon chili powder

Instructions:

Step 1: Rinse the quinoa under cold water in a fine mesh strainer to remove any bitterness.

Step 2: In a medium saucepan, bring the 2 cups of water or vegetable broth to a boil. Add the quinoa, cover, and reduce heat to low. Cook for about 15 minutes, or until all the liquid is absorbed and the quinoa is fluffy.

Step 3: While the quinoa is cooking, prepare the vegetables. Dice the red bell pepper, avocado, and red onion. Chop the cilantro. Set aside.

Step 4: In a small bowl, whisk together the lime juice, olive oil, salt, and pepper. Add ground cumin and chili powder if using, to create a dressing.

Step 5: Once the quinoa is cooked, transfer it to a large mixing bowl and let it cool for a few minutes.

Step 6: Add the drained and rinsed black beans, diced red bell pepper, chopped red onion, and cilantro to the bowl with the quinoa.

Step 7: Drizzle the dressing over the quinoa and vegetable mixture. Gently toss everything together until well combined.

Step 8: Gently fold in the diced avocado to the mixture, being careful not to mash it.

Step 9: Taste and adjust seasoning with additional salt, pepper, lime juice, or spices as needed.

Step 10: Serve the quinoa and black bean bowl at room temperature or chilled. It can be enjoyed on its own or as a side dish.

Nutritional Note: This quinoa and black bean bowl is packed with plant-based protein, fiber, and healthy fats. Quinoa is a complete protein, containing all nine essential amino acids, which is beneficial for muscle repair and growth. Black beans are high in fiber, supporting digestive health. Avocado provides healthy monounsaturated fats, which are heart-healthy and can help with the absorption of other nutrients.

Recipe 9: Turkey and Avocado Sandwich

Ingredients Needed:

- 2 slices of whole grain bread

- 4 ounces of sliced turkey breast (preferably organic)

- 1 ripe avocado

- 1 tablespoon of Dijon mustard (or to taste)

- Lettuce leaves (such as romaine or butter lettuce)

- 2 slices of tomato

- Salt and pepper to taste

Instructions:

Step 1: Toast the two slices of whole grain bread lightly in a toaster until they are just golden brown. This step is optional but provides a nice texture to the sandwich.

Step 2: While the bread is toasting, cut the avocado in half, remove the pit, and scoop out the flesh into a small bowl.

Step 3: Mash the avocado with a fork until it's creamy but still has some chunks for texture. Season the mashed avocado with a pinch of salt and pepper to enhance its flavor.

Step 4: Spread the Dijon mustard evenly on one slice of the toasted bread. The mustard adds a tangy flavor that complements the turkey and avocado beautifully.

Step 5: Lay the sliced turkey breast on top of the mustard-spread bread slice. If you prefer, you can slightly overlap the slices for a fuller sandwich.

Step 6: Place the lettuce leaves over the turkey slices. Lettuce not only adds a crunch to your sandwich but also provides a fresh, leafy flavor.

Step 7: Add the tomato slices on top of the lettuce. Tomatoes add a juicy, slightly acidic taste that balances the creaminess of the avocado.

Step 8: Spread the mashed avocado on the second slice of toasted bread. This will be the top layer of your sandwich, adding a rich, buttery texture and flavor.

Step 9: Carefully place the avocado-spread slice on top of the tomato slices, avocado side down, to complete your sandwich.

Step 10: Cut the sandwich in half if desired. This makes it easier to handle and eat, especially if you're on the go.

Nutritional Note: This turkey and avocado sandwich is a balanced meal option, offering a good mix of protein, healthy fats, and fiber. Whole grain bread provides complex carbohydrates for sustained energy, while turkey is a lean source of protein that supports muscle health. Avocado is rich in heart-healthy monounsaturated fats and fiber, making this sandwich a nutritious choice for those looking to support their thyroid health and overall well-being.

Recipe 10: Lentil Soup

Ingredients:

- 1 tablespoon olive oil
- 1 medium onion, diced
- 2 cloves garlic, minced
- 1 carrot, peeled and diced
- 1 stalk of celery, diced
- 1 cup dried lentils (green or brown), rinsed
- 4 cups vegetable broth
- 1 teaspoon ground cumin
- 1/2 teaspoon ground coriander
- 1/2 teaspoon salt
- 1/4 teaspoon black pepper
- 1 bay leaf
- 2 tablespoons tomato paste
- 2 cups spinach leaves, roughly chopped

- Juice of 1/2 lemon
- Optional: Fresh cilantro or parsley for garnish

Instructions:

Step 1: Heat the olive oil in a large pot over medium heat. Add the diced onion and sauté until it becomes translucent, about 5 minutes.

Step 2: Add the minced garlic, diced carrot, and celery to the pot. Cook, stirring occasionally, for another 5 minutes, or until the vegetables start to soften.

Step 3: Stir in the rinsed lentils, vegetable broth, ground cumin, ground coriander, salt, black pepper, and bay leaf. Increase the heat to bring the mixture to a boil.

Step 4: Once boiling, reduce the heat to low, cover the pot, and simmer for about 25-30 minutes, or until the lentils are tender.

Step 5: Remove the bay leaf from the pot. Stir in the tomato paste and chopped spinach. Continue to simmer for another 5 minutes, or until the spinach is wilted and the soup has thickened slightly.

Step 6: Stir in the lemon juice and adjust seasoning with additional salt and pepper if necessary.

Step 7: Serve the lentil soup hot, garnished with fresh cilantro or parsley if desired.

Nutritional Note: Lentils are an excellent source of protein, fiber, and essential nutrients that support thyroid health, including selenium and iron. This soup is not only nourishing but also comforting, making it a perfect choice for a healing diet.

Chapter 15:
Recipes and Meal Planning Tools

15.2 EASY RECIPES FOR DINNER

Recipe 11: Baked Salmon with Asparagus

Ingredients Needed:

- 2 salmon fillets (6 ounces each)

- 1 tablespoon olive oil

- Salt and pepper to taste

- 1 bunch asparagus, ends trimmed

- 1 lemon, sliced into rounds

- Optional: Fresh dill or parsley for garnish

Instructions:

Step 1: Preheat your oven to 400°F (200°C). Line a baking sheet with parchment paper for easy cleanup.

Step 2: Place the salmon fillets on the prepared baking sheet. Brush each fillet with olive oil and season generously with salt and pepper.

Step 3: Arrange the asparagus around the salmon fillets. Drizzle the asparagus with the remaining olive oil and season with salt and pepper. Toss lightly to ensure the asparagus is well-coated.

Step 4: Lay lemon slices over the salmon fillets. This adds moisture and a zesty flavor to the salmon as it bakes.

Step 5: Bake in the preheated oven for about 12-15 minutes, or until the salmon is cooked through and flakes easily with a fork. The exact cooking time may vary depending on the thickness of the fillets.

Step 6: While the salmon and asparagus are baking, prepare your garnish. If using, chop the fresh dill or parsley.

Step 7: Once the salmon and asparagus are done, remove from the oven. Sprinkle the fresh dill or parsley over the top for added flavor and a pop of color.

Step 8: Serve immediately. For a complete meal, consider adding a side of quinoa or a fresh salad.

Nutritional Note: Salmon is rich in omega-3 fatty acids, which are essential for reducing inflammation and supporting thyroid health. Asparagus is a great source of fiber, folate, and vitamins A, C, and K. Together, this meal is not only delicious but also packed with nutrients beneficial for those managing Hashimoto's.

Chapter 15:
Recipes and Meal Planning Tools

Recipe 12: Chicken Stir Fry with Vegetables

Ingredients:

- 1 boneless, skinless chicken breast (about 6 oz), thinly sliced

- 2 tablespoons soy sauce (low sodium preferred)

- 1 tablespoon sesame oil

- 1 tablespoon olive oil

- 1 cup broccoli florets

- 1/2 bell pepper, sliced (color of your choice)

- 1/2 onion, sliced

- 1 carrot, julienned

- 2 cloves garlic, minced

- 1 teaspoon ginger, grated

- Optional: 1 tablespoon honey (for a touch of sweetness)

- Optional: sesame seeds and sliced green onions for garnish

Instructions:

Step 1: In a mixing bowl, combine the thinly sliced chicken breast with soy sauce and sesame oil. Let it marinate for at least 15 minutes to enhance the flavor. If you have time, marinating for an hour or more in the refrigerator can make the chicken even more flavorful.

Step 2: Heat olive oil in a large skillet or wok over medium-high heat. Once hot, add the marinated chicken slices. Stir-fry until the chicken is fully cooked and no longer pink in the center, about 5-7 minutes. Remove the chicken from the skillet and set aside.

Step 3: In the same skillet, add a bit more olive oil if necessary. Add the broccoli florets, sliced bell pepper, sliced onion, and julienned carrot. Stir-fry the vegetables for about 3-4 minutes until they are just tender but still crisp.

Step 4: Add the minced garlic and grated ginger to the skillet with the vegetables. Stir-fry for another minute until the garlic and ginger are fragrant.

Step 5: Return the cooked chicken to the skillet with the vegetables. If you're using honey, add it now. Stir everything together and cook for another 2-3 minutes, ensuring the chicken and vegetables are well coated with the sauce and honey if used.

Step 6: Taste and adjust seasoning if necessary. You can add a little more soy sauce or a dash of salt if needed.

Step 7: Serve the chicken stir-fry hot. Garnish with sesame seeds and sliced green onions if desired.

Step 8: This dish pairs beautifully with steamed rice or quinoa for a complete meal.

Nutritional Note: This chicken stir-fry is packed with protein from the chicken and a variety of vitamins and minerals from the colorful vegetables. Using low-sodium soy sauce helps manage salt intake, and the sesame oil adds healthy fats that are beneficial for hormone balance and inflammation reduction.

Recipe 13: Spaghetti Squash with Marinara Sauce

Ingredients Needed:

- 1 medium spaghetti squash
- 2 tablespoons olive oil
- Salt and pepper to taste
- 1 jar (24 ounces) marinara sauce (choose a low-sugar, gluten-free option if necessary)
- 1 teaspoon dried Italian herbs (basil, oregano, thyme mix)
- Optional: Fresh basil leaves for garnish
- Optional: Grated Parmesan cheese (or a dairy-free alternative)

Instructions:

Step 1: Preheat your oven to 400°F (205°C). Line a baking sheet with parchment paper for easy cleanup.

Step 2: Carefully cut the spaghetti squash in half lengthwise with a sharp knife. Scoop out and discard the seeds and stringy flesh with a spoon.

Step 3: Drizzle the olive oil over the cut sides of the spaghetti squash. Season with salt and pepper to taste.

Step 4: Place the squash halves cut-side down on the prepared baking sheet. Roast in the preheated oven for 40-50 minutes, or until the flesh is tender and easily shreds with a fork.

Step 5: While the squash is roasting, heat the marinara sauce in a saucepan over medium heat. Stir in the dried Italian herbs. Reduce the heat to low and let it simmer until the squash is ready, stirring occasionally.

Step 6: Remove the squash from the oven and let it cool for a few minutes until it's safe to handle. Use a fork to scrape the inside of the squash, creating spaghetti-like strands.

Step 7: Divide the spaghetti squash strands among plates. Top with the warm marinara sauce.

Step 8: Garnish with fresh basil leaves and grated Parmesan cheese if desired.

Step 9: Serve immediately, offering a comforting and nutritious meal that aligns with your health goals.

Nutritional Note: Spaghetti squash is a low-calorie, low-carb alternative to traditional pasta, making it an excellent choice for those managing Hashimoto's and seeking weight loss. It's also rich in vitamins A, C, and B, along with minerals like potassium and magnesium. Pairing it with a homemade or high-quality store-bought marinara sauce adds flavor without the added sugars and unhealthy fats found in many commercial varieties.

Recipe 14: Stuffed Bell Peppers

Ingredients Needed:

- 4 large bell peppers (any color)
- 1 lb ground turkey or a plant-based alternative
- 1 tablespoon olive oil
- 1 small onion, diced
- 2 cloves garlic, minced
- 1 cup cooked quinoa or rice
- 1 can (15 oz) black beans, drained and rinsed
- 1 cup corn (frozen or canned)
- 1 teaspoon ground cumin
- 1/2 teaspoon chili powder
- 1/2 teaspoon salt
- 1/4 teaspoon black pepper
- 1 cup shredded cheese (optional, use a dairy-free cheese if necessary)
- 1/2 cup salsa, plus extra for serving
- Fresh cilantro for garnish (optional)

Instructions:

Step 1: Preheat your oven to 375°F (190°C). Prepare a baking dish by lightly greasing it with olive oil or cooking spray.

Step 2: Slice the bell peppers in half from top to bottom, and remove the seeds and membranes. Place the bell pepper halves in the prepared baking dish, cut side up.

Step 3: In a large skillet over medium heat, add 1 tablespoon of olive oil. Once hot, add the diced onion and cook until translucent, about 3-4 minutes.

Step 4: Add the minced garlic to the skillet and cook for an additional minute until fragrant.

Step 5: Add the ground turkey or plant-based alternative to the skillet. Cook, breaking it apart with a spoon, until it is no longer pink, about 5-7 minutes.

Step 6: Stir in the cooked quinoa or rice, black beans, corn, ground cumin, chili powder, salt, and black pepper. Cook for another 2-3 minutes until everything is well combined and heated through.

Step 7: Remove the skillet from heat. If using, stir in the shredded cheese and 1/2 cup of salsa until everything is evenly mixed.

Step 8: Spoon the mixture into each bell pepper half, pressing down slightly to pack them well. Cover the baking dish with aluminum foil.

Step 9: Bake in the preheated oven for about 30 minutes. Remove the foil, and if desired, top each stuffed pepper with a bit more cheese. Return to the oven, uncovered, for an additional 10 minutes, or until the peppers are tender and the cheese is melted and bubbly.

Step 10: Let the stuffed bell peppers cool for a few minutes before serving. Garnish with fresh cilantro and serve with extra salsa on the side.

Nutritional Note: This recipe provides a balanced meal with protein from the turkey or plant-based alternative, fiber from the quinoa or rice and black beans, and a variety of vitamins and minerals from the bell peppers and corn. It's a nutrient-dense option that supports overall health, including thyroid function.

Recipe 15: Zucchini Noodles with Pesto

Ingredients Needed:

- 2 medium zucchinis

- 1 cup fresh basil leaves

- 1/4 cup pine nuts

- 2 cloves garlic

- 1/2 cup extra-virgin olive oil

- 1/4 cup grated Parmesan cheese (use a dairy-free alternative if necessary)

- Salt and pepper to taste

- Optional: Cherry tomatoes for garnish

- Optional: Additional grated Parmesan cheese for serving

Instructions:

Step 1: Begin by making the zucchini noodles. Use a spiralizer to turn the zucchinis into noodles. If you don't have a spiralizer, you can use a vegetable peeler to create long, thin strips. Set the noodles aside.

Step 2: Toast the pine nuts in a small skillet over medium heat. Stir frequently to prevent burning, until they are golden brown and fragrant, about 3-5 minutes. Remove from heat and allow to cool.

Step 3: In a food processor, combine the basil leaves, toasted pine nuts, and garlic cloves. Pulse until coarsely chopped.

Step 4: With the food processor running, slowly add the olive oil in a steady stream. Continue to process until the mixture is smooth.

Step 5: Transfer the pesto mixture to a bowl. Stir in the grated Parmesan cheese. Season with salt and pepper to taste. Adjust the consistency by adding more olive oil if necessary.

Step 6: In a large bowl, combine the zucchini noodles and pesto. Toss until the noodles are evenly coated. Let sit for a few minutes to allow the flavors to meld and the noodles to soften slightly.

Step 7: If using, halve cherry tomatoes and add them to the bowl. Toss gently to combine.

Step 8: Serve the zucchini noodles with pesto in bowls. If desired, garnish with additional grated Parmesan cheese and a few fresh basil leaves.

Nutritional Note: Zucchini noodles are a low-carb, nutrient-dense alternative to traditional pasta, making them an excellent choice for those managing Hashimoto's. The pesto provides healthy fats from the olive oil and pine nuts, which can help support hormone balance and reduce inflammation.

15.3: 7-Day Meal Plan Examples

Day 1:

- **Breakfast:** Simple Avocado Toast topped with sliced tomatoes and a sprinkle of hemp seeds for added protein.

- **Lunch:** Grilled Chicken Salad with mixed greens, cucumbers, cherry tomatoes, and a balsamic vinaigrette.

- **Dinner:** Baked Salmon with Asparagus, seasoned with lemon, garlic, and dill. Serve with a side of quinoa.

Day 2:

- **Breakfast:** Quick Oatmeal with Berries, a dollop of almond butter, and a drizzle of maple syrup.

- **Lunch:** Veggie Wrap with Hummus, spinach, shredded carrots, and sliced red bell peppers in a whole wheat tortilla.

- **Dinner:** Chicken Stir Fry with Vegetables including broccoli, bell peppers, and snap peas over brown rice.

Day 3:

- **Breakfast:** Easy Greek Yogurt Parfait with a layer of mixed berries, a sprinkle of granola, and a dash of cinnamon.

- **Lunch:** Quinoa and Black Bean Bowl with avocado, salsa, and a squeeze of lime.

- **Dinner:** Spaghetti Squash with Marinara Sauce, topped with sautéed mushrooms and a sprinkle of nutritional yeast.

Day 4:

- **Breakfast:** Basic Smoothie Bowl with spinach, banana, mixed berries, and almond milk, topped with sliced almonds and chia seeds.

- **Lunch:** Turkey and Avocado Sandwich on whole grain bread with lettuce and mustard.

- **Dinner:** Stuffed Bell Peppers with a mixture of ground turkey, cooked brown rice, diced tomatoes, and spices.

Day 5:

- **Breakfast:** Classic Scrambled Eggs with spinach and mushrooms, served with a side of whole grain toast.

- **Lunch:** Lentil Soup with carrots, celery, and tomatoes, seasoned with thyme and rosemary.

- **Dinner:** Zucchini Noodles with Pesto and cherry tomatoes, topped with grilled chicken strips.

Day 6:

- **Breakfast:** Smoothie with spinach, avocado, banana, protein powder, and almond milk.

- **Lunch:** Mixed Greens Salad with sliced strawberries, almonds, and goat cheese, drizzled with a vinaigrette.

- **Dinner:** Baked Cod with a side of roasted sweet potatoes and steamed green beans.

Chapter 15:
Recipes and Meal Planning Tools

Day 7:

- **Breakfast:** Overnight Oats with chia seeds, almond milk, and topped with fresh mango and coconut flakes.

- **Lunch:** Chickpea Salad with cucumbers, tomatoes, olives, feta, and a lemon-olive oil dressing.

- **Dinner:** Grilled Eggplant and Zucchini Stacks with marinara sauce and a sprinkle of parmesan cheese.

Each meal is designed to provide a balanced intake of nutrients, support thyroid function, and reduce inflammation. Remember to adjust portion sizes according to your individual needs and preferences. Drinking plenty of water throughout the day and incorporating gentle exercise into your routine can further enhance your well-being.

Made in United States
Troutdale, OR
07/20/2025